YOUR HEALTHY HEART

YOUR HEALTHY HEART

A GUIDE TO HOW THE HEART WORKS AND HOW TO KEEP IT HEALTHY

CHRISTIAAN BARNARD

WITH PETER EVANS

Macdonald

A **Macdonald** BOOK

First published in Great Britain in 1985
by Macdonald & Co (Publishers) Ltd
London & Sydney

A member of BPCC plc

British Library Cataloguing in Publication Data
Barnard, Christiaan
    Your healthy heart.
    1. Heart – Diseases – Prevention
    I. Title   II. Evans, Peter, *1940-*
    616.1′205   RC682

    ISBN 0-356-10524-5

This book was devised and produced by
Multimedia Publications (UK) Limited.

Editors: Caroline Morrow Brown
            Andie Oppenheimer
Design: John Youé & Associates
Picture Research: Mira Connolly
Production: Judy Rasmussen, Hugh Allan

Origination by Reprocolor Llovet, Barcelona
Typeset by Rowland Phototypesetting (London) Ltd
Printed and bound in Italy by New Interlitho SpA

Macdonald & Co (Publishers) Ltd
Maxwell House
74 Worship Street
London EC2A 2EN

Contents

Preface   7

PART I   THE HEART: how it works and what goes wrong   9

Introduction to Part I   11

Chapter 1   **The Early Years**   12

Chapter 2   **Accidents of Birth:** congenital heart disorders   48

Chapter 3   **Acquired Heart Disease:** diagnosing dangers   64

Chapter 4   **Treating Acquired Heart Disease**   88

Chapter 5   **Heart Attack and Counterattack**   120

Chapter 6   **Cardiac Research and Technology**   144

PART II   KEEPING HEALTHY   153

Introduction to Part II   155

Chapter 7   **Controlling Stress**   156

Chapter 8   **How to Stop Smoking:** a plan that works   180

Chapter 9   **Diet and Keeping Fit**   188

Index   219

Acknowledgements   223

Picture Credits   224

Preface

I have often been asked why I write books and articles on medical subjects for the general public, because surely a little knowledge is a dangerous thing? A little knowledge can indeed be dangerous but I consider that no knowledge is even more dangerous.

Medicine has only recently emerged from the Dark Ages, where prescriptions were written in Latin so that the patients would not know what they were taking. People are now hungry for knowledge about how their bodies work and what can go wrong with them. I have always believed that patients should be accurately informed about their medical problems – the treatment of an illness is teamwork, and the most important member of this team is the patient.

Since I performed the first heart transplant using a human donor, there has been a clamour for more information about the heart, that simple little pump which has been surrounded by so much mystique over the ages. I have had the privilege to address thousands of people all over the world on various aspects of heart disease, and the interest generated by these meetings has been so intense that I decided to write this book, *Your Healthy Heart.*

When my medical career started, the management of heart disease mainly consisted of monitoring patients by taking their pulse and blood pressure. The only special investigation was a chest X-ray and the only treatments were digitalis, diuretics and bed-rest. Today, we have the fantastic facilities of the intensive care unit and scores of drugs to choose from. When I was a junior doctor, the surgical treatment of heart disease was merely an attempt to correct lesions around the heart. Today there is *no* heart condition that cannot either be corrected or improved by surgical intervention.

In *Your Healthy Heart,* I have relived this exciting period of my medical career and have attempted to bring the reader up-to-date on the treatment of heart disease. But even more important, I have outlined the ways that many of these potentially fatal conditions can be prevented.

Christiaan Barnard

Part I

The Heart:
how it works
and what goes wrong

Introduction

In all the medical dictionary, surely there can be no word more evocative than the word 'heart'.

The heart it is that keeps us alive, pumping blood around the body like some biological dynamo throbbing away ceaselessly day and night; it is a source of vitality without which we quickly cease to function. The heart provides the driving force for the body. And it is the heart that we imagine to control our deepest feelings. Cupid's arrow finds its way to the heart to stir the emotions of love and affection. The rock star or movie actor becomes a 'heart throb', capturing the attention of millions of idolizing fans. Or perhaps we are 'sick at heart' at the sight of pain and suffering in the world. Of course, the idea that the heart is the seat of the emotions is a misleading piece of folklore, just as the symmetrical, bright red heart on the Valentine's Day card owes little to anatomical reality.

Over the centuries people have built up quaintly inaccurate notions about the heart's qualities and functions, probably because there seemed to be some logic in linking the centre of our physical being – the organ that pumps life-giving forces round the body – with the core of our feelings. The ardent suitor whose pulse quickens and whose heart pounds when he catches sight of his beloved seems to exhibit a connection between mind and body. And poets and playrights have been quick to turn this into a metaphor about the very nature of emotion, which is both triggered off by and reflected in the pounding, fluttering, leaping and breaking of the heart.

By contrast, when I recently had the chance to talk to some Bushmen of the Kalahari I found that this vital organ, so surrounded by Western mystique, holds no special meaning for them. When I asked them what the heart symbolized to them, they said simply that it was a pump that pushed blood around the body; they had observed it working as the life-blood flowed from a hunted antelope. It is odd that it took us, in so-called advanced societies, so long to acknowledge something so simple.

Chapter 1
The Early Years

So powerful was our tradition of regarding the heart to be the spiritual as well as the physical centre of our existence that it led to a feeling that the heart was somehow sacrosanct when compared with other organs of the body: this untouchable organ was definitely not to be violated by a surgeon.

Indeed, the great physicians of antiquity believed the heart to be a delicate natural mechanism that, once interfered with, could not be repaired. Two thousand years ago Hippocrates wrote that injuries to the heart were sure to be fatal, while Aristotle too considered that 'The heart alone of all viscera cannot withstand serious injury'. Somewhat later, Galen studied the wounds received by gladiators and concluded that a sword or spear to the heart was sure to cause death if it reached the ventricles – a belief echoed in the eighteenth century by Boerhaave, who was similarly convinced of the mortal dangers attendant to piercing wounds.

By and large this was the medical orthodoxy for around 20 centuries, although a few observant individuals had, on occasions, noticed that not everyone with a heart injury actually died from it. Moreover, from early in the seventeenth century there is a report of two autopsies in which undeniable evidence of previous cardiac injury was found, even though neither of the deceased had met their deaths as a result of this. This finding was confirmed later in another report: at the autopsy a scar had been found in the heart of a man who had been pierced by a sword some four years before. The heart, it seemed, could be touched without killing a person – indeed, it seemed to be positively robust!

It was, however, some time before surgeons began seriously to build on these early observations and to contemplate deliberately operating on people with heart disease or injury. There were exceptions, such as Napoleon's famous surgeon Baron Dominique-Jean Larrey, who in 1829 successfully managed to drain fluid off the heart of a soldier who had suffered a stab wound. After the operation, he ventured to suggest that his fellow doctors had taken 'too grave a view of the effects of wounds' in this hitherto untouchable area, but his fellow surgeons were far from quick to respond. In fact, it was not until the late 1860s that the medical profession began to consider surgery as a serious option in the treatment of cardiac disease – and even then fairly reluctantly. the heart was still beyond the 'last frontier', which few were keen to cross. As late as 1896 Stephen Paget

This is the heart of Andreas Roscuer, who was stabbed while drinking in October 1682. The wound was not fatal, and the healed scar was revealed at the autopsy some years later, after he had died from other causes.

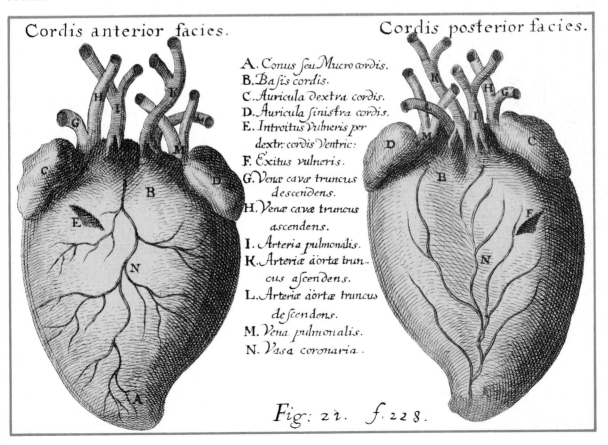

Cordis anterior facies.　　　Cordis posterior facies.

A. *Conus seu Mucro cordis.*
B. *Basis cordis.*
C. *Auricula dextra cordis.*
D. *Auricula sinistra cordis.*
E. *Introitus vulneris per dextr. cordis Ventric:*
F. *Exitus vulneris.*
G. *Venæ cavæ truncus descendens.*
H. *Venæ cavæ truncus ascendens.*
I. *Arteria pulmonalis.*
K. *Arteriæ aörtæ truncus ascendens.*
L. *Arteriæ aörtæ truncus descendens.*
M. *Vena pulmonalis.*
N. *Vasa coronaria.*

Fig: 22.　f. 228.

could affirm that 'no new methods, no new discovery, can overcome the natural defects that attend a wound of the heart'. Around the same time, the celebrated Viennese surgeon Christian Albert Theodor Billroth warned, 'Let no man who hopes to retain the respect of his medical brethren dare operate on the human heart'. This was, said Billroth, 'prostitution of the surgical art, if not downright madness'.

As the twentieth century drew nearer, then, the heart was still regarded as out-of-bounds by most of the medical profession – but, significantly, not by all. One of the most fascinating stories in the whole of medical history was beginning to take shape. Bit by bit, the 'forbidden territory' would slowly be opened up by courageous and farsighted doctors, whose skill and intelligence would be matched only by their remarkable determination.

JOURNEY TO THE CENTRE OF THE HEART

For me, the single most important date in the early history of heart surgery is 9 September 1896, for it was on that day that a 22-year-old man, Wilhelm Justus, was operated on by Ludwig Rehn. Rehn, a German surgeon, successfully stitched up a wound in Justus' heart which went on to heal perfectly, thus demonstrating beyond all doubt that the human heart could actually be handled while a person was alive – and the patient could live to tell the tale to his or her grandchildren. The touch of the scalpel, the intrusion of the suturing needle, the probing of the doctor's finger – none of these could any longer be dismissed as rash or foolhardy attempts to tamper with nature to the detriment of the patient. At last surgeons were beginning to take their rightful place in the struggle to fight diseases of the heart.

Rehn's success produced a fresh note of optimism among surgeons. Up to that time the vast majority of surgical interventions had been purely experimental. Animals such as dogs had been used in the study of, for example, the action of the heart's very special valves, or rabbits in the testing out of the effects of suturing wounds. But now that a *human* heart had been at the centre of the action things were different – as I

The evolution of surgical techniques, 1646 to 1986.
a) A German engraving of 1646.
b) Surgery at Charing Cross Hospital, London, 1900.
c) A patient's view, 1986.

was to discover, in a rather similar context, several decades later when I performed the first heart-transplant operation. When you do something for the first time you learn a great deal, both about the operation and about yourself, and your confidence increases with every new thing you undertake.

Audacious surgeons

And so it was in the wake of Rehn's operation on Herr Justus. Papers were written in medical journals suggesting that surgery could be the answer for diseases that had previously been virtually untreatable. In 1897 one Dr. Tuffier successfully treated a case of cardiac arrest (when the heart-pump just stops) by applying massage, while elsewhere there was talk of surgically correcting defects in the heart's valve mechanisms. Sir Lauder Brunton, a leading surgeon of his day, wrote to the medical journal, *The Lancet*, suggesting that it might be possible to widen a narrowed valve-opening by surgical means, and pointing out that he had come to this opinion after experimenting with cats in the laboratory. A week later he was verbally chastized for being the champion of such a dangerous procedure – cats or no cats – while others wondered if the valve-opening would stay open after surgery, or revert to its unhealthy constriction. But for all the initial opposition the tide was undoubtedly on the turn.

Over the next ten years or so enthusiasm for heart surgery, especially in connection with the relief of valve blockages, built up steadily. In those pioneering days, from the turn of the century to around the outbreak of the First World War in 1914, this enthusiasm was primarily directed towards animal experiments. In Europe and the USA medical researchers used laboratory animals to try out various techniques for correcting valve deformities; these, though far from perfect, helped to spread the notion that soon such operations might safely be performed on humans.

War wounds

In the event, however, things did not speed ahead quite so rapidly as one might have anticipated. There was a bit of a hiatus with the coming of the First World War, when surgeons were preoccupied not so much with furthering

Many new surgical techniques were developed as a result of knowledge gained during the First World War.

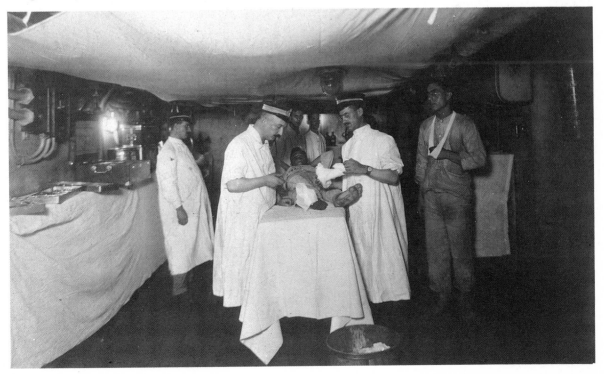

the experimental measures initiated in peace-time as with coping with the wounds to the heart incurred on the battlefield. However, the very fact that doctors were forced to operate on so many heart wounds was both highly instructive and encouraging for the future. It became obvious that the heart was indeed a rugged organ which would tolerate far more manipulation and 'interference' than most people had realized. Although many of the medical records of those war years have been lost, the documents that survive show that the success rate among heart-wound operations was very high. After the war, this fact gave even greater impetus to experimental work on the development of cardiac surgery for the disorders of peacetime.

The first great landmark in the post-war phase was in may 1923 when Cutler, Levine and Beck operated on an 11-year-old girl whose life was threatened by a defective heart valve. Having delicately worked their way in through the heart chamber known as the left ventricle, they managed, using a special surgical knife, to enlarge the valve-opening by separating the flaps or cusps which had become fused as a result of inflammation. As it happens, the patient, although surviving the operation and indeed going on to live for a further four-and-a-half years, did not show a marked improvement in her condition after the operation. Cutler and his team tried to improve matters during four more operations over the next two years, but with little success. However, we should not undervalue their efforts. After centuries of mystery, the heart, that *terra incognita* of the human body, had at last been penetrated by the scalpel, had continued to function, and had even been revisited by the surgeon for later attempts to improve its performance.

Quick thinking and new discoveries
In 1925 Henry Souttar, a surgeon whose invention, 'Souttar's Eyeless Needle', is still in use in operating theatres around the world, carried out the first successful mitral stenosis (blockage of the mitral valve) operation on a patient called Lily Hine, who had been given a mere six months to live. It was an extraordinary operation, and it illustrated a feature of surgery that has often struck me as fundamental: the

need for thinking quickly 'on your feet' and adapting to the circumstances of the moment.

Souttar had begun the operation with the intention of opening up the blocked valve with a surgical instrument, just as Cutler had done. But, during the course of the operation, he changed his mind and instead used his index finger, passing it through the valve orifice, where it met with no resistance: the blockage was cleared. Souttar then began to sew up the incisions he had made. Suddenly a snag occurred. The suturing gave way and he had to work fantastically fast in order to complete the proceedings within a reasonable space of time. In total, the operation had lasted one hour – not lengthy by today's standards, perhaps (I can remember many seven-, even eight-hour sessions in the theatre), but it was a long time in 1925.

With this successful operation Souttar had fully justified a prediction he had earlier made in the *British Medical Journal*:

Incisions can be made in its [the heart's] chamber, portions of its structure can be excised and internal manipulations carried out without the slightest interference in its action and there is ample evidence that wounds of the heart heal as readily as those in any other region.

In the wake of the Lily Hine success, other valve operations were carried out during the 1920s by surgeons elsewhere. There were just a handful, though, and unfortunately all the patients died. So what might have been a flood turned out to be a mere trickle, with most of the medical establishment being reluctant to promote further operations of this type. Souttar himself was, for all his undoubted skill, never sent any more mitral-valve cases to treat, the general feeling being that such operations were still just on the fringes of the reputable.

In other words, although the tide seemed to be about to turn so far as cardiac surgery was concerned, there was no spectacular attempt by surgeons to force the pace. Heart injuries were still their principal interest. The correction of mechanical defects would have to wait more than 15 years before the next major steps could be taken: the modern assault on the diseased and

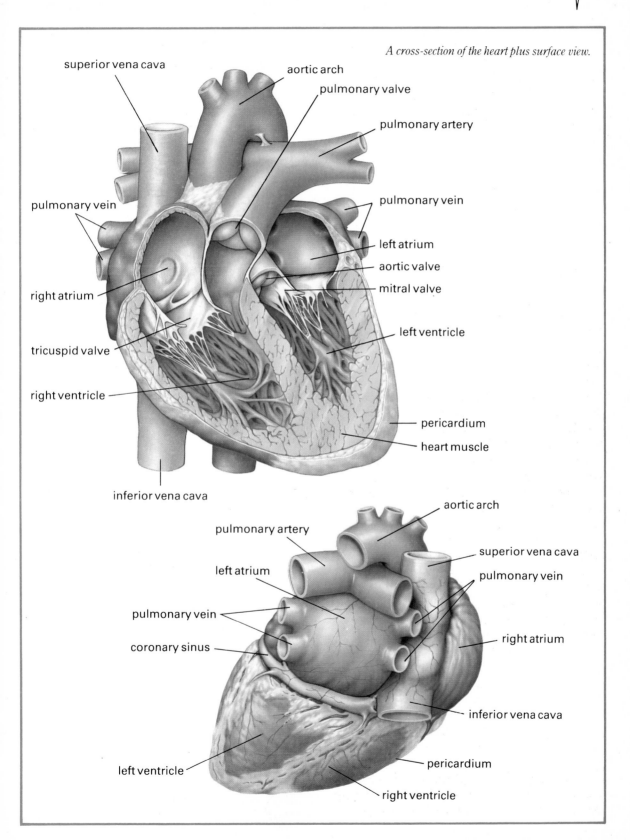

A cross-section of the heart plus surface view.

superior vena cava

aortic arch

pulmonary valve

pulmonary artery

pulmonary vein

pulmonary vein

left atrium

aortic valve

mitral valve

right atrium

left ventricle

tricuspid valve

right ventricle

pericardium

heart muscle

inferior vena cava

aortic arch

pulmonary artery

superior vena cava

left atrium

pulmonary vein

pulmonary vein

coronary sinus

right atrium

left ventricle

inferior vena cava

pericardium

right ventricle

malfunctioning heart. However, before we move on to watch this dramatic story unfold, perhaps we should 'freeze the frame' here in the mid-1920s to take a closer look at the heart itself. What does it do, how does it do it, and what can go wrong with it?

A MATTER OF THE HEART: INSIDE THE PUMPING ROOM

Clench your fist and you have a rough idea of the size of your own heart.

The heart is a truly remarkable piece of natural engineering: day and night, whether we are sleeping deeply or exercising violently, the mere 250–350 g of heart muscle continues to act as our vital pump, maintaining the circulation of blood through our bodies with a smoothness and coordination that any mechanical engineer could only marvel at, and certainly never hope to replicate in a man-made system.

The mechanics

Before we look more closely at the route taken by the circulating blood, I want to dwell on this exquisite biological pump – a mechanism that has fascinated me for well over 30 years.

The heart is roughly conical in shape, and mostly hollow. It consists of four chambers, two on each side, separated by a wall called the *septum*. The top chamber on both sides is the *atrium*, a Latin word that means literally an entrance hall. Indeed, the right and left atria are, as it were, the reception areas for the blood, where it enters to prime the two pumping units. These are the chambers below, called the *ventricles*, which have thicker muscular walls perfectly designed to expand and contract powerfully in order to send the blood on its way to all parts of the body.

Blood travels from each atrium into its respective ventricle through a one-way valve; these valves prevent blood, once in the ventricles, from flowing back into the atria. The valve allowing blood to flow from the left atrium into the left ventricle is known as the *mitral valve*, so-called because it has two flaps and looks a little like a bishop's pointed headpiece – a mitre. The valve between the right atrium and the right ventricle is the *tricuspid valve*, so-called because

it consists of three flaps, or 'cusps'. There are two further valves. One is the *aortic valve*, which leads from the left ventricle to the aorta, the main distributing artery, and prevents blood leaking back into the left ventricle once it has been pumped through. The other is the *pulmonary valve*, leading from the right ventricle into the pulmonary artery, and preventing blood from leaking back once it has been pumped towards the lungs.

I well remember when this arrangement of valves and chambers was first introduced to me in my student days. We were given the usual anatomy lectures illustrated by charts, diagrams and blackboard sketches. Then we went off to pore over similar schematic representations in our textbooks; in addition, there was a three-dimensional plastic model of a heart that we could handle. Before long I felt I knew what the human heart looked like inside and out.

Anatomy classes and textbooks can be very misleading, though. If you are looking at a picture of the heart, you see only that – the heart. But once the chest cavity is opened up in the

Blood circulation

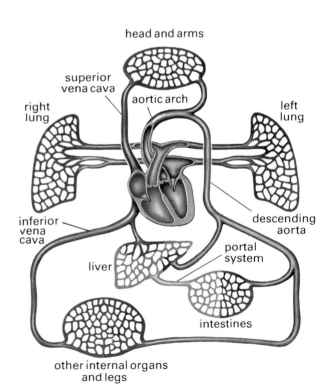

operating theatre what you see is very different from the illustrations. The organs do not stand out in stark contrast and relief, one from another. Nor is the heart a tidy-looking, strongly outlined object in glowing colours, with each region and its attendant blood vessels thoughtfully picked out in contrasting shades and hues. Suddenly, the textbook gets left behind as you begin to see the body's central pumping room as a living, breathing, natural entity.

The circulation

You begin to marvel at the way it continues to beat 100 000 times a day, continuously pumping about 5 litres of blood per minute around the circulatory system, handling some 7000 litres of blood every 24 hours. That means that, in the average lifetime, nearly 200 million litres are circulated around the body.

The basic route of the blood's remarkable journey is this. Fresh blood (i.e., blood saturated with oxygen (O_2) and bright red in colour) is pushed from the left ventricle through the aortic valve into the aorta. It then flows through the arteries to all parts of the body, where it supplies the various tissues with essential oxygen and other nutrients. Once these life-giving nutrients have been expended, leaving in their stead carbon dioxide (CO_2), water and other waste-products, the blood, now dark purplish-red (it is often called 'blue' or venous blood) flows through the veins back to the heart, entering the right atrium (or receiving area). It then passes through the tricuspid valve into the right ventricle; from here it is pumped through the pulmonary valve into the pulmonary artery, which leads to the lungs. In the lungs the blood is oxygenated and water and CO_2 are extracted; it then flows through the pulmonary veins to the left atrium, ready to begin the cycle again.

There is, then, a strict route taken by the blood: from the body via the veins to the right side of the heart, from there to the lungs, from the lungs to the left side of the heart and from there back to the body via the arteries. This is where those one-way valves become important, ensuring that the blood does not seep back. And, of course, in order to maintain sufficient driving force the heart has to keep going – the body cannot wait for fresh supplies of oxygenated

Arteries, veins and capillaries

blood. The wastes soon become toxic unless they are removed and replaced by fresh oxygen.

The blood is carried by three kinds of vessels: *arteries*, which take blood from the heart to the body's tissues and lungs; *veins*, which carry it on its return journey to the heart; and *capillaries*, which act as link roads, as it were, connecting the smaller arteries to the smaller veins. (Note that, while normally veins carry 'blue' blood and arteries carry oxygenated blood, the pulmonary vessels are the exception – the pulmonary vein carries red blood and the pulmonary artery carries 'blue'.) Thus when an artery reaches a muscle, for example, it will branch out into tiny capillaries so that the blood can enter the muscle itself. After being deprived of its oxygen and loaded with waste products, the blood then leaves the muscle through a similar network of capillaries which then join up at a vein. Think of the capillaries as the smallest twigs of a tree, carrying nourishment from the main boughs and larger branches to all the leaves.

Keeping the beat

The heartbeat is regulated by a crescent of specialized cells situated in the upper part of the

Thicker than water . . .

No one did more to advance the cause of scientific medicine than the English doctor William Harvey (1578-1657). He made history by showing that blood is constantly on the move through the body, so breaking with the accepted wisdom handed down by Galen, who believed that the heart acted as a low-temperature oven to keep the blood warm and that the movement of blood was not like water through a pipe, but was comparable to the ebb and flow of a tidal seepage.

Harvey's key contribution was his treatise on the movement of the heart and blood in animals, *Exercitatio Anatomica de Motu Cordis et Sanguinis in Animalibus.* In it he demonstrated with admirable scientific clarity that the heat beats by muscular contraction, squeezing the blood out of its interior into the arteries through the one-way valves, and returning it to the heart in the veins. He was able to show that what came back to the heart was indeed the same blood as that which had left it, not a newly manufactured quantity, as others had thought. In short, he concluded that blood was recycled.

Although Harvey accurately described the phenomena of circulation and blood pressure, he did not have a microscope (the instrument had yet to be invented), and so could not identify the exact means by which blood pressure was maintained – the fine capillaries.

The four to six litres of blood in our bodies accounts for one-fourteenth of our total body weight. Blood consists mostly of fluid. This fluid portion is *plasma,* a pale brown, sticky liquid containing, among other things, proteins, salts, cholesterol, glucose, lipids and hormones. All these need to be transported from one part of the body to another, by the blood.

The plasma also carries the various blood cells. Red cells contain haemoglobin, which is a molecule capable of picking up, carrying and delivering oxygen. Haemoglobin is very similar in its molecular structure to chlorophyll in plants, which suggest an evolutionary link between the two. White cells, or leukocytes, are larger than red cells and are responsible for fighting infection. There are also special cells for causing the blood to clot: the platelets, or thrombocytes. In any cubic millimetre of blood there are approximately five million red cells, 10 000 white cells and around 250 000 platelets.

William Harvey

a) *A human-to-animal blood transfusion carried out in 1679. At that time doctors had no knowledge of blood groups.*

b) *Relative proportions of the formed elements of the blood.*

c) *A portion of a blood clot, showing filaments of fibrin around a trapped red cell.*

a

plasma

white cells

red cells

platelets

b

c

The pumping cycle of the heart

A *The atria are full, with ventricle walls relaxing, all valves closed. The small arrows from the superior and inferior vena cavae, and from the pulmonary veins indicate flow from the body's system.*

B *The atria emptying into the ventricles, the tricuspid and mitral valves having floated open. The aortic and pulmonary valves are closed. The small arrows indicate slow blood movement.*

C *Atrial systole now takes place. Blood passes rapidly into the ventricles from the contracting atria, with the aortic and pulmonary valves still closed. Full flow is indicated by larger arrows.*

D *Ventricular systole is now initiated. Back pressure from blood in the ventricles closes the tricuspid and mitral valves. The aortic and pulmonary valves are about to snap open from mounting pressure within the*

ventricles. The atria start to refill from the vena cavae and pulmonary veins. Back pressure and filling of the atria are indicated by appropriately-sized arrows. Commencement of muscular activity in the ventricle walls is indicated by the ridged condition of the inner surfaces.

E *Ventricular systole now takes place. Ventricle walls close in causing blood to flow through the aortic and pulmonary valves, which are now fully open, into the body's system. The tricuspid and mitral valves are still closed. The atria continue to fill. Full flow is indicated by larger arrows.*

F *Ventricular systole is now completed and the aortic and pulmonary valves are about to snap shut; the ventricle wall muscle is beginning to relax, indicated by the smoother condition of the inner surfaces. The atria continue to fill.*

*This open-heart illustration shows the electrical control and conducting system of the heart. **A** is the left atrium, **B** the left ventricle, **C** the aorta, **D** the pulmonary artery, **E** the right atrium, **F** the right ventricle, **G** the pacemaker, and **H** the atrioventricular node.*

The entire pumping system of the heart relies on modified tracts of muscle fibres. These contract like normal muscle cells but they also transmit impulses like nerve cells.

Electrical signals travel from the pacemaker along specially modified muscle fibres. These stimulate the atria to contract, squeezing blood through the tricuspid and mitral valves and into the ventricles below. These atrial signals travel at a speed of 1m/second (3ft/second). As soon as they reach the atrioventricular node they trigger off more electrical signals; these travel down more specialized muscle fibres – at a speed of 5m/second (17ft/second) – into the walls of the ventricles. The ventricles then contract, from bottom to top, forcing blood into the aorta and the pulmonary artery.

The delay in conduction of impulses between the atria and ventricles means that blood has left the atria, entered the ventricles and the valves have shut properly between them, before the powerful ventricular pumping occurs.

right atrium. Measuring 2.5 cm by 3–4 mm, this group of cells is called the *sino-atrial node*. By a mechanism not yet understood, the cells of the node spontaneously discharge a tiny electrical current 60 to 70 times per minute. This current spreads along the walls of both atria to another node, the *atrio-ventricular node*, in the bottom left-hand corner of the right atrium, close to the septum between the two ventricles. From here the signal passes along a set of nerve fibres called the Bundle of His, down the inside of both ventricles before it finally turns back up the outer walls of the ventricles, so that the electric current is spread from the inside of the wall to the outside. When heart-muscle cells are stimulated by electricity they contract, and so the effect of this process is to initiate the heartbeat.

WHAT GOES WRONG

The heart, although seemingly complex, really has only three components – its muscles, its valves and its nervous system. Any affliction of the heart is a disease affecting either one, or a combination, of these parts.

Diseases affecting the heart muscle

Among the main killers in the Western world is coronary artery disease, which causes impairments in the flow of blood to nourish the heart muscle itself. It is important not to forget that the heart is largely muscle, of a special kind called *myocardium*, which like any other muscle has to get a constant supply of fresh blood in order to function properly. The main arterial diseases are *atheroma*, the slow deterioration of arteries in which fatty deposits are laid down in the inner lining, and *arteriosclerosis*, the thickening and hardening of the usually supple arterial walls – remember, though, that while these commonly affect the coronary arteries, and therefore lead to disease of the heart muscles, they are primarily diseases of the arteries, not of the heart itself.

The effects of these diseases are pronounced

A photomicrograph of heart tissue showing the Bundle of His and the myocardium.

Cross-section of a normal artery (above).

Cross-section of an artery wall that has become thick and hardened (above).

A view of the fatty deposits known as atheroma (below).

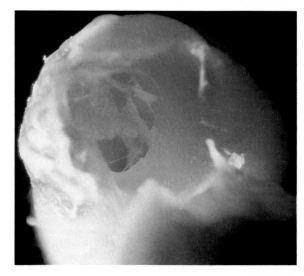

and dangerous. If an artery is clogged with a fatty lining, like the spout of a kettle with 'fur', blood-supply is impaired or even blocked altogether. Or the deposits may cause cracks and distortions in the normally smooth arterial wall, whereupon blood may form clots (thromboses) which stem blood-flow. Or the wall of the artery may be weakened so that it begins to bleed or haemorrhage. Or it may just become unduly tough (hardening of the arteries): without elasticity, blood vessels are inefficient carriers of fluid, like a garden hose that has become brittle. Or, finally, the circular muscle-coat of an artery may go into spasm, causing undue constriction and impeding blood-flow.

The faster the heart pumps, the greater the blood-flow through the coronary arteries. If that flow is being impeded, however, we feel a rapidly developing pain in the centre of our chest and a tightening or constriction across it called angina, which is really a warning that things may get serious unless we ease up the pressure. If we do not do so, the heart is forced to continue its violent activity with an inadequate supply of blood (ischemia) and the pain continues, leading to permanent damage of the heart muscle.

The heart muscle can also be damaged by viral infections, such as by the Coxsackie viruses, or by overwork as a result of leaking valves. Sometimes the heart muscle can be abnormal without apparent cause, as occurs in conditions called cardiomyopathies – these affect all age groups, but are fortunately fairly rare.

Diseases affecting the heart valves

The second category of heart problems concerns the valves, which, like the parts of any machine, can malfunction in a variety of ways. As we have seen, blood must follow a programmed route and not flow back and forth. Once it has passed a certain point, on it must go, to return only when it has been full-cycle through the circulatory system. This is where the one-way action of the various valves is of paramount importance. Valve disease can give the heart surgeon many hours of repair work before the valves are set back in working order.

Contrary to popular belief, the commonest heart disease, taken worldwide, is either narrowing or leakage of the valves caused by rheumatic heart disease. Rheumatic heart disease is the sequel to rheumatic fever, which in turn results from an initial streptococcal infection (streptococci are a type of bacteria). The disease produces inflammation in the heart muscle and valves and can be quite severe, especially among children and teenagers. Fortunately, the incidence of rheumatic fever has declined in those countries where antibiotic treatments are readily available – but that still leaves many parts of the world with a young population at risk.

Valves can be impaired in other ways – as a result of syphilis, for instance – or a patient may simply have a congenital deformity of the valves, or may have acquired this as a sequel to coronary thrombosis. Whatever the cause, the effects may prevent the valve from opening fully (*stenosis* – 'constriction'), or may stop it closing properly, allowing blood to leak back after it has come through, a condition known as *incompetence*. Both conditions present the heart with an unhealthily large workload. It has to pump harder to force blood through a stenosed valve or to maintain proper flow if blood is seeping back.

There is a further complication for people with a malfunctioning valve: they can sometimes succumb to infection of the valves, *endocarditis*. The infection is usually caused by bacteria and is often a consequence of receiving dental treatment. So, before they have their teeth treated, susceptible patients should take a precautionary dose of antibiotics.

Defects of the nervous system

The third type of problem is caused by failure of the heart's nervous system. As we have seen, the rhythm of the heart is dictated by a fascinating electrical, chemical and muscular timekeeping mechanism. This too can go wrong, producing disorders of rhythm or *arrhythmias*. The pathways along which the signal from the pacemaker cells is sent must be kept open and clear, since otherwise the message may become

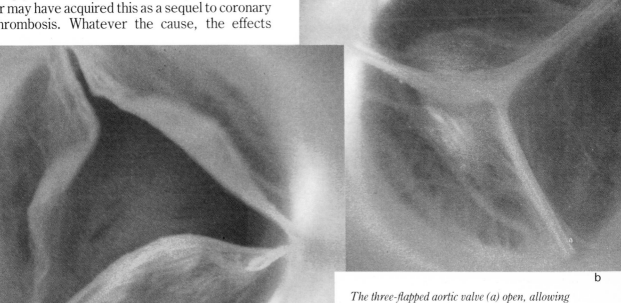

The three-flapped aortic valve (a) open, allowing blood to be pumped through, and (b) closed.

garbled. If the route is diseased this is exactly what happens: the muscle cells receive instructions to beat either too quickly (*tachycardia*) or too slowly (*bradycardia*). In addition, irregularities such as extra beats and atrial fibrillation can occur. Some can be controlled by a regime of drugs, while others benefit from an artificial pacemaker – still others can be prevented altogether.

If, for some reason, the sino-atrial node fails, any other part of the heart can take over its function and keep the heart contracting – albeit at a slower rate. This is seen dramatically in a condition called atrio-ventricular block where, although the heartbeat originates normally in the right atrium, it cannot be conducted down the Bundle of His and so the ventricles produce their own 'node'. The condition stabilizes with the atria beating at their usual 60 to 70 beats per minute and the ventricles beating at a much slower rate, say 40 to 50 beats per minute. Since the ventricular contractions produce the pulse which is felt at the wrist or neck, this condition can be detected by a slowing of the pulse-rate. If the slowing is severe enough to cause symptoms such as blackouts, the ventricles will require help to speed them up a little, and a pacemaker will probably be inserted.

THE ROAD TO OPEN-HEART SURGERY

Ever since medicine began, people have been trying – vainly, until recent times – to give effective treatment for serious heart complaints. The modern assault on the heart began at about the time that Hitler was undertaking his assault on the rest of the world. The year was 1938 and the surgeon was Robert Gross of the Harvard Medical School in Boston. Gross was one of a number of doctors who had been anxious to attempt the surgical treatment of congenital cardiac defects. He had been encouraged by progress made in the important (and often overlooked) field of anaesthesia, which was enabling the surgical team to maintain greater control over the patient's respiration while the chest was open. For example, in London Ivan Magill gave pre-war surgeons the ability to remove all or part of an infected or cancerous lung while the patient remained satisfactorily

An X-ray showing a pacemaker in place.

anaesthetized. This also gave the surgeons a chance to familiarize themselves with prolonged surgery in the region of the heart. Moreover, great advances had been made in stitching blood vessels together.

Confident that his patients were being well looked after by the anaesthetists, Gross decided to attempt an operation on a condition that had been first described by the great physician, Galen, 800 years before – patent ductus arteriosus. His patient was a seven-year-old child suffering from this inborn defect, whereby blood leaks from the aorta to the pulmonary artery because a channel or duct has remained open ('patent') after birth instead of closing up a few hours or days after the lungs have begun to function. This results in a shunt of blood between the aorta and pulmonary artery, which floods the lungs and puts strain on the left-hand side of the heart; if the condition is untreated the child becomes and remains an invalid. It is estimated that, of all the congenital abnormalities of the heart and surrounding vessels, patent ductus accounts for 17 out of every 100 cases, so you can see why Gross's planned operation had considerable importance for future generations of unfortunate children.

To cut a long story short, Gross managed to tie off the duct, the operation was a brilliant success, and the news of this major advance spread quickly. Today the operation is routine, but I can remember when it was a life-and-death matter, with many dying on the operating table because we could not control the bleeding.

EARLY BYPASS SURGERY

While Gross and others were developing the surgery for closing an unwanted opening, other surgeons were working on the complementary problem of getting rid of dangerous obstructions. There are two ways of doing this. Either you can break through or widen the blockage, or you can attempt to bypass the obstruction by providing an alternative route for the blood to follow. It is, I suppose, the difference between picking your way through a traffic jam or turning off into a side road to rejoin the main highway later on. During the late 1930s and early 1940s, Professor Alfred Blalock of Johns Hopkins University in the USA investigated this second strategy, developing a technique for linking together (anastomizing) main blood vessels. In 1944 this painstaking research and imaginative clinical application reached its high spot when the bypassing method was used to alleviate one of the severe congenital defects which cause what is popularly known as a 'blue baby'. Why 'blue'? Well, normally bright-red oxygenated blood is pumped from the heart to the rest of the body, but sometimes a child is born with one or a group of defects that allow unoxygenated blood to get into the system instead. Thus the body, instead of receiving freshly invigorated blood, is supplied with blood lacking in oxygen and character-

istically very dark purplish-red in colour. This gives the skin a blue tinge. The less oxygen, the bluer the baby.

First attempts at a 'blue baby' operation

The 'blue baby' Blalock operated on in 1944 had a constriction of the pulmonary valve and an opening between the ventricles. He decided that the blueness would be reduced if he could link up a main artery in the aorta straight to the pulmonary artery; in other words, create a 'shunt'. It would be only a partial correction of the defect but, if it were successful, the child should be able to live a normal, healthy life.

That, at least, was the theory, but Blalock knew very well that the technical problems were formidable and the uncertainties many. Not only was the actual surgery itself very intricate, but the patient was very young. Could a child survive this major assault on its heart? What would be the effect on the aorta, from which he was going

The 'blue baby' operation as performed by Blalock. The left subclavian artery is connected to the left pulmonary artery.

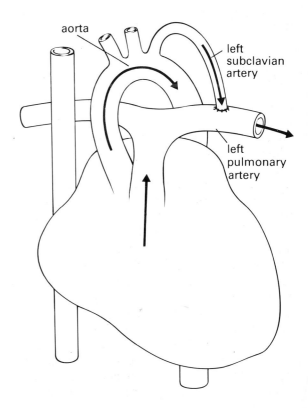

aorta

left subclavian artery

left pulmonary artery

The pioneering work of Blalock and Gross gave babies like this the chance of life.

permanently to 'borrow' a blood vessel? Then there was the perennial problem that faced all heart surgery – time. The projected 'blue baby' operation was likely to take at least 30 minutes, during which time the blood-supply to the lungs would be stemmed. What would this do to the lungs themselves? A lot of questions and a life, not to mention the fortunes of heart surgery in general, hung on this operation.

The relief and excitement when it succeeded were immense. Immediately a great many children would reap the benefit but, perhaps just as important, the cardiac surgeon became a specialist in his own right, and taken his rightful place within the surgical mainstream.

Getting to the heart of the matter

Up until the 1940s, surgeons were really working *around* the heart, rather than within it. Throughout the rest of the 1940s a variety of new avenues were explored to correct defects inside the heart, building on the long-awaited successes of Blalock and others. As an alternative to the bypassing of a narrowed pulmonary valve, Thomas (now Sir Thomas) Holmes Sellors managed, in 1947, to alleviate the obstruction by operating on the valve itself, and approached the problem of narrowed mitral valves by breaking the obstruction with dilators introduced into the heart.

This was the period of closed-heart surgery: all of these heroic efforts to improve the heart and circulatory system were hampered because the surgeons were having to work 'blind'. It was still impossible to undertake profoundly intensive procedures within the heart for the simple reason that it could not be isolated from the rest of the body for long enough to allow the surgeon to do his job. Without some artificial pause in the heart's natural activities, there was little chance of being able to carry out sophisticated surgery.

The long-term answer was, of course, to develop machines that would take over the heart's work for long periods in the operating theatre. Before that, however, we used what now seems a rather crude method of buying time, 'borrowed', so to speak, from the winter habits of certain animals. It was the clinical equivalent of hibernation.

GAINING TIME

By cooling down the body it is possible to slow down its metabolic rate in roughly the same way as hibernating animals change their metabolisms for winter. Indeed, there have been reports of individuals lost in the snow who have remained in a state of suspended animation in conditions of extreme cold, being apparently 'dead' when found but coming back to life when warmed up again. Could a state of low body temperature – hypothermia – be deliberately induced for long enough to allow corrective surgery to be performed?

Wilfred Bigelow in Canada, using cooling on anaesthetized animals, had managed to slow the heart-beat down from 180 to 25 beats a minute, and had noted how breathing and other bodily rates had also dropped. Indeed, in 1950 Bigelow saw a great future for cooling, estimating that it would allow organs to be excluded from circulation for long periods, so that surgeons could operate on a bloodless heart without recourse to external pumps, and perhaps allow transplantation of organs. In 1952 he was able to cool a body to around 30°C and show that this arrested circulation for ten minutes or so without causing brain damage. The way seemed clear for a whole range of open-heart procedures.

Within months, John Lewis and his colleagues at the Minnesota Medical School (where I was later to work and study) put theory into practice by using hypothermia in an operation to close a hole between the atria in the heart of a five-year-old girl. She was cooled down in special rubber cooling blankets and the blood-flow to the heart was stopped by clamping the two major veins bringing blood back to the heart. This allowed surgeons five-and-a-half minutes to open the heart, stitch the defect, and close up the incision. Then the clamps were removed, the blood flowed again and the young patient was warmed up to normal temperature. She recovered completely.

Encouraged by this success, other doctors

A tiny baby being cooled down with cold water and ice to enable a life-saving operation to be performed.

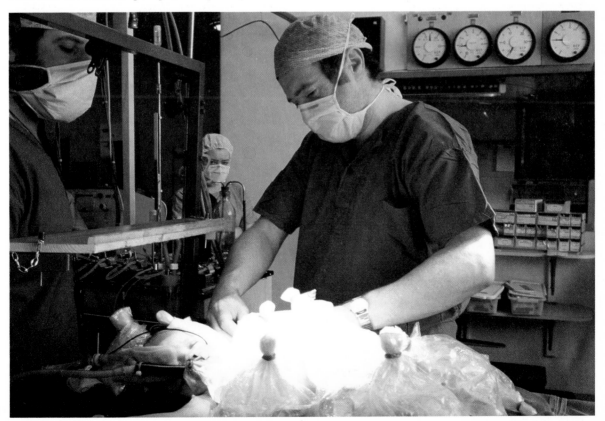

Sanne is pictured here in 1976 when she was six months old and weighed five kilos. Her body was being cooled down with cold water and ice so that open-heart surgery could be performed. The operation took about thirty-five minutes, and within four days she was on her mother's knee having her first meal from a bottle.

pushed ahead with ways of cooling and rewarming the body. Warming was sometimes done by passing a short-wave current through coils in a blanket wrapped round the cold patient or simply by putting the patient into a warm bath. For cooling, some adopted the technique of passing the blood out from the arteries through a cooling coil and returning it to the body via the veins. Others used special drugs which allowed more rapid cooling. But by far the most popular cooling method was to immerse the patient in a cold-water bath spiked with plenty of ice. The anaesthetized patient would be given the cooling bath and then rushed onto the operating table so that the surgeons could do their work within what was still a very limited space of time.

The whole method was, however, far from satisfactory. To slow the metabolism sufficiently to arrest brain damage, very low temperatures are required. But, if the body temperature is reduced to less than 30 to 32 °C, *fibrillation* (irregular twitching) of the heart muscle and death can result. At these temperatures, the circulation can be arrested for only seven to ten minutes before irreversible damage to the central nervous system is incurred. So time was still at a very great premium, and any complex manipulations just could not be attempted.

The real breakthroughs would become possible only when surgeons could be supported by a machine that would pump blood through the body and through an artificial 'lung' that would supply it with essential oxygen. With an efficient extra-corporeal circulator and oxygenator there would be no need to complete intricate surgery in a matter of minutes; there would be none of the risks that had been experienced using hypothermia.

One of the first viable heart–lung machines was developed by the US professor of surgery, John Gibbon. Together with his wife, he built an experimental machine which was used successfully on cats. But it was to be more than 15 years before Gibbon's heart–lung apparatus was wheeled into the operating theatre for use in heart surgery on a human patient, so great were the technical difficulties in developing it, not to mention the sometimes less-than-enthusiastic attitudes of the medical profession.

However, mechanical imitations of the respiration process are still feeble compared with the perfect biological mechanisms contained within the mammalian form. This intricate, silent, unbelievably efficient arrangement, containing lungs with a gas-exchange surface larger than a tennis court, will never be replicated in our or our children's lifetimes. We still have much to learn.

A dormouse hibernating. The idea of lowering the body's metabolic rate by cooling was developed from observations on hibernating animals.

Gibbon's oxygenator

Gibbon's extra-corporeal oxygenator consisted of two pumps, one pushing blood through the artificial lung, the other through the body's arteries. The oxygenator (also known as the film oxygenator) was an arrangement of stainless steel layers which made up a large surface area over which oxygen was blown. The blood was pumped over these screens, where it could pick up oxygen to transport to the arteries while releasing carbon dioxide – its main waste product – at the same time. Once in the arteries the pumped blood had, of course, to flow freely but without being squeezed, which would have damaged the structure of the blood cells, while in the machine there was the added problem of blood sticking to the various pipes and junctions and clogging up the smooth mechanism. Gibbon managed to resolve these difficulties in the laboratory, and in 1954 used his machine to aid him in an operation on an 18-year-old girl suffering from an atrial septal defect. She was connected up to it for 45 minutes, for 25 of which the mechanical device completely took over the function of the heart. Open-heart surgery with

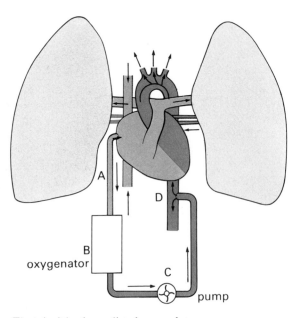

The principle of a cardiopulmonary bypass.
The venous blood is collected from the upper and lower great veins (A), flows into the oxygenator (B), then through a pump (C), and back into a large systemic artery at a convenient site (D).

the heart–lung machine had taken its first decisive step.

At the same time as artificial extra-corporeal cardiorespiratory systems were in their infancy, another time-seeking technique was being developed. Instead of passing the blood of the patient through a machine, why not use another human circulatory system – a biological life-support method that avoided all the problems associated with man-made pumps, valves, pipes and tubes? Animal experiments by Anthony Andreason in the UK had demonstrated that such a cross-circulation arrangement could work: the functioning of one animal's heart and lungs could temporarily be taken over by a second animal, then restored, without harming either borrower or lender. Could this be extended to heart patients during operations?

Lillehei's cross-circulation technique

The man who was to provide an answer to that question was my teacher, one of the great characters in the story of heart surgery, the controversial and brilliant Walton Lillehei of the University of Minnesota. Himself a cancer sufferer who had survived, Lillehei lived by the philosophy of trying to give his own patients a chance, whatever the loading of the dice against them. Building on Andreason's ideas, Lillehei brought cross-circulation techniques to such a level of development that in 1955 he felt able to put them into practice with a cardiac operation in which the circulation of a father was linked to that of his son. Although this particular operation was unsuccessful, in that the patient died two weeks later, the actual circulatory demonstration had been extremely convincing. Lillehei went on to perform more than 50 operations using cross-circulation, including 'blue baby' patients among his many subsequent successes. No one claimed that here was *the* answer to the problem of finding time for long operations, but it was at least a useful alternative to cooling and to the early versions of the heart–lung machines.

How did cross-circulation work? The idea was very simple. A catheter was inserted into a vein in the groin of the patient. Blood from here was pumped by means of an external pump into a vein in his father's (the donor's) groin. From there the patient's blood was circulated through the

The principle of the screen oxygenator.

donor's system and pumped and oxygenated by his heart and lungs. Another catheter was inserted into an artery in the donor's groin, and from here oxygenated blood was artificially pumped into a corresponding artery in the patient's body, thus providing crucial life-support while the heart was isolated for surgery. Both donor and patient had to be treated with anticoagulants in order to prevent clotting while the cross-circulation was taking place.

A PERSONAL VIEW

And it was at this juncture that I, a young South African doctor, had the good fortune to be awarded a scholarship to study and work in the USA. The year was 1956 and I went to a thriving centre for advanced heart-surgery techniques – the University of Minnesota – the very place where John Lewis had made enormous strides in using hypothermia, and Lillehei was applying his

formidable mind to cross-circulation and heart–lung machines. When I arrived at Minnesota there occurred one of those quite unforeseen chances that seem at first to be insignificant, but it was to change the course of my life.

My appointment was as a general surgeon, not as a heart specialist. Indeed, at that time general surgery was what I wanted to do, with particular leanings towards correcting defects or injuries to the oesophagus. As it happened, though, my lab was situated alongside that of Dr. Vincent Gott, who was deeply immersed in developing heart–lung machine technology. Passing by his room I would catch sight of the complicated arrangements of hardware, and occasionally stop to talk to Vincent about his work. After a time, I began to get more than a little interested in what was going on in this newly emergent field of open-heart surgery – an interest that was fuelled from time to time when Gott would ask me to help him connect up some of the various pipes

The author at work at the Groote Schuur Hospital, Cape Town, South Africa.

and tubes on his elaborate machine. Hooking up those connectors hooked me. I asked to be transferred to heart surgery . . .

Looking at history, even quite recent history, can be deceptive because one tends to think that events and ideas all drop into place in neat chronological order, one following the other like a well-behaved crocodile of schoolchildren. In reality the picture is always more complicated. During my early days as a heart surgeon in the USA, there was never a question of one technique replacing another overnight. Two or several methods might be practised at any one time, often by the same doctor, until he was sure that technique A could be superseded by technique B because the latter had shown itself to be superior.

In the mid-1950s, for instance, the heart–lung machine had not established a monopoly over the hypothermal and cross-circulation methods for open-heart operations. Nor, indeed, had the major successes in open-heart surgery proved to the whole of the medical profession that this was a branch of their art worthy of intensive development. On one occasion Lillehei presented a paper in Minneapolis describing his marvellous work with 'blue baby' operations. As he finished, a cardiologist who was a proponent of a rival method stood up and said, 'The tragedy of this kind of operation, Dr Lillehei, is that some of your patients survive. Now others will try their hand, and who knows what sort of disastrous results they'll have.' Ten years later I was to hear much the same remark made about heart transplants, and I knew then how Lillehei must have felt: being condemned, not for ineptitude, but for competence. Such are the paradoxes of practising medicine.

Trailblazing . . . or cooling
But the opponents of open-heart surgery belonged to a dwindling minority, a fast-disappearing dinosaur species among doctors in general. I was too caught up in the prospects afforded by these operations to care much about the doubters, for those were great pioneering days. We were still carrying out cooling operations, dipping patients in icy baths, working at breakneck speed on the operating table and then rewarming. I worked on an alternative hypothermia technique, intragastric cooling, based on the fact that the stomach has a particularly rich blood supply. The idea was to anaesthetize an experimental animal and pass down into its stomach a small balloon. Cold water was pumped down the tube into the balloon,

thereby cooling the stomach's blood-supply and so having an overall blood-cooling effect on the body. This would enable cooling while the chest was being opened and rewarming while the chest was being closed, reducing operating time and hence the risk. As we came to build the machine we ran into a problem, though. Where could we find small, slim balloons that would be watertight within the animal's stomach? Suddenly the solution came to me: we could try using rubber condoms. After all, they are manufactured to resist a certain amount of fluid pressure and they are about the right size. Someone was despatched to purchase some contraceptive sheaths and these were duly tried out. The brainwave worked, so the laboratory sent in a requisition for a large stock of rubber condoms, purely, of course, for scientific and medical use . . .

Ultimately, intragastric cooling did not become widely used in heart surgery, but there was an interesting spin-off. Cooling the stomach reduces not only temperature but also acidity levels, so my technique was taken up and used for treating stomach ulcers.

Improving cross-circulation

Alongside our work on cooling the programme of research into better cross-circulation procedures continued. In particular, we were trying to make such operations safer for the donor, who ran the constant risk of infection. Finally, however, human donors had to be abandoned when one mother, whose circulation was married up to that of her baby, developed severe brain damage after an air bubble blocked a vital artery. If a biological oxygenator were to be used, an alternative to a human being had to be found. For a while the lungs of animals such as dogs were used, but it eventually became clear that the only really satisfactory method of controlled oxygenation was by machine. Gibbon had already shown that such a device could be built, although his apparatus had the twin disadvantages of great complexity and considerable expense. Were there any other ways of putting oxygen into the blood of a patient?

The bubble oxygenator

In Minnesota there was a young researcher named Richard De Wall who had begun to tackle the problem in the early 1950s. As I was making my debut as a heart surgeon and researcher, De Wall's 'bubble oxygenator' was just coming into service. Basically the device consisted of a tubular chamber into which the venous blood was pumped to be mixed with large oxygen bubbles; the refreshed blood was then pumped on into an artery. Although the principle of the bubble oxygenator seems straightforward enough, in practice there were formidable problems to be overcome. For one thing the entry of a bubble of oxygen into the bloodstream could be fatal, so, before the oxygenated blood could be circulated, all airlocks had to be removed, a problem which De Wall tackled by interposing a de-bubbling chamber in the machine at the top of the column of blood as well as introducing a special anti-foam chemical into the system to break down the bubbles. Even with these refinements, heart operations using this machine could be harrowingly dramatic affairs. The blood would often simply bubble out of the machine in vast quantities, sometimes reducing the volume of blood available to dangerous levels, so that the surgeons had to rush frantically before the blood ran out. I can still remember the tensions, because at that time I had the job of supervising the oxygenator in the theatre. Such crises also created a terrific mess all over everything, including the surgeons. Even when anti-foam came into use there were still dangers: too little anti-foam and the blood would bubble out; too much and it would produce tiny emboli of anti-foam in the blood, and these could block a patient's circulation. In short, a good deal of trial and error, of experimentation and clinical risk, was involved. But bit by bit De Wall's machine was refined and improved to the point where we could draw on a comparatively inexpensive, effective and uncomplicated oxygenator for major heart surgery.

The membrane oxygenator

Another route, later to be developed to a high degree of sophistication, was the membrane oxygenator. This was a mechanical attempt to mimic the way the gas-exchange of carbon dioxide and oxygen takes place in the lungs. In both lungs and machine a semipermeable membrane acts as a one-way sieve, whereby

A modified Lillehei-type bubble oxygenator in use in 1957 at Guys Hospital, London.

oxygen molecules (O_2) are diffused through into the blood and carbon dioxide molecules (CO_2) are diffused out into the airsacs of the lungs. In theory this method should have been ideal, as it reduced the risk of bubbles of air being introduced into the patient's circulation, but it was extremely difficult to find an adequate membrane.

As far as I was concerned, I felt at the time that I had been let into heart surgery on the ground floor. My whole ambition as a doctor had been to *do* things, to make a positive, visible and practical contribution to the health and welfare of the patient. Surgery offered the right sort of outlet for my aspirations. Now that open-heart surgery was beginning to emerge, it seemed almost pre-ordained that this should become my speciality. I could make the sort of direct interventions I favoured in what many had regarded as sacred territory. Heart–lung machines had given me and others the means to tread on hallowed ground.

For the next ten years, until that fateful day in 1967 when I performed the first human transplant, I played my part in the general development of modern heart surgery, working on a variety of the classic problems of cardiology. The important point was that we now had the *time* to correct complex defects of all kinds: rather than minutes, we had hours.

The matter of diagnosis

These developments precipitated, indeed demanded, corresponding improvements in the absolutely vital fields of diagnostic and monitoring techniques. Before anything can possibly be attempted by way of treatment for a patient, it is imperative to assess the extent of his problem. In addition to a verbal account of symptoms and outward physical signs of disease, we need to 'see' the inside of the body and how the heart is performing before we can think of making surgical incisions. Later on I shall be discussing the use of such invaluable tools as X-rays and the electrocardiograph – ECG – but here we should

The principle of a bubble oxygenator.

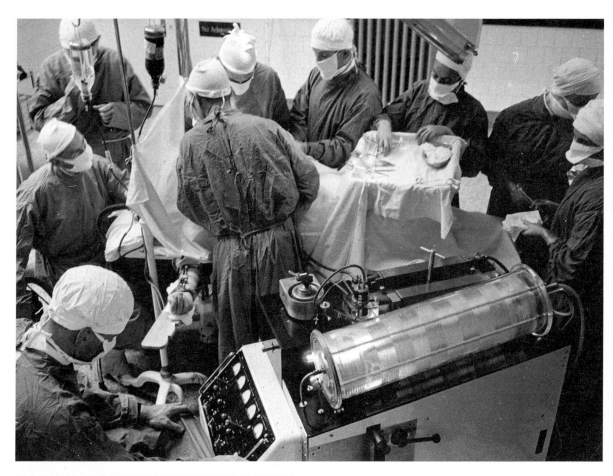

A heart-lung machine in use in 1956 (above),
compared to the modern machinery
used today (below and left).

perhaps dwell a little on the pioneers of diagnostic science.

Think, for example, of a young and, to his fellow-doctors, rash individual called Werner Forssman, who in 1929 carried out an experiment that verged on the foolhardy – or so

A prototype ECG machine developed by the Cambridge Instrument company in 1911 (above).

Einthoven's original electrocardiograph, built by him in his physiological research laboratory, weighed 800 pounds, occupied parts of two rooms, and required five people to operate (top).

it seemed at the time. Forssman was convinced that it was possible to study the function of the heart by direct instrumentation. His original idea was to find an efficient way of delivering drugs to the circulatory system in an emergency, which meant, he reasoned, getting them into the heart very promptly. But how to do this? Using corpses in the hospital mortuary Forssman practised inserting fine tubes – catheters – into a vein near the elbow and threading this into the right side of the heart. He became so skilful at this that he then decided to take the dramatic step of trying it out on himself. He inserted a catheter into his own arm, pushed it carefully back, back into the heart, and then walked along the corridor to the X-ray department to confirm that he had indeed inserted the catheter into his right atrium. He predicted that here was a means, not just of getting drugs to the site of action very rapidly, but also of studying the function of the heart.

His optimism was borne out. Doctors in the UK and the USA developed this catheterization procedure so that it became, if not routine, at least standard practice when it was not clear from other diagnostic methods in what way the heart was defective. Today high technology has taken over, and catheters are treated with radio-opaque dyes so that they can be monitored visually on television screens. But it took the courage of a dedicated doctor who put his money where his mouth was to get it all started.

FIRST THOUGHTS ON TRANSPLANTS

A surgeon does what he does within the context of other people who are working or have worked in the same or related fields. Without the research of Pasteur, for example, it is difficult to imagine Fleming and Florey giving the world penicillin. And where would any heart doctor be today if Harvey and others had not helped to lay the foundations of our understanding of the basic circulation of the blood?

As a young surgeon I began fully to appreciate this interdependence in medicine when my thoughts started to take a turn towards a different kind of surgery: not just trying to correct the defects in a heart, but replacing a dying heart with one in good health. I knew that

as long ago as 1912 the great French surgeon Alexis Carrel had been awarded a Nobel Prize for his trailblazing work with animals, demonstrating that transplantation surgery was possible, at least in principle. And, like other cardiac surgeons, I had of course read of the intriguing experiments made by a Russian, Vladimir Demikhov, who had succeeded in transplanting an animal heart that beat in parallel with the recipient's own heart for ten days before the creature died. And in 1956 a surgeon had succeeded in grafting the head of one puppy onto the neck of another, demonstrating that the intricate procedures necessary were feasible.

Was transplantation of vital organs, including the heart, no longer one of those comic-strip fantasies? Was it technically and practically conceivable?

While I turned over this enticing prospect in my mind, I knew that there were some pretty big problems to be resolved. Supposing we could use a heart–lung machine to take over a patient's circulation and respiration while we gave him or her a new heart, where was this organ to come from? Presumably a recently deceased donor, but here there were two major difficulties. Firstly, the donor would have to die in the right place and at the right time, which seemed too much of a lucky coincidence. Secondly, and this was perhaps a more fundamental point, the human body is designed not to accept foreign tissue but to reject it. There are exceptions – the cornea in the eye, cartilage in the limbs, and, of course, blood of matching groups can be switched from one individual to another. But with the heart and other parts of the body the immune system acts as a permanent sentry guard, ever alert and ready to oust invaders.

Rejection was a major barrier, but I was sure that it was not insurmountable. Had not a successful kidney graft been performed in 1954? Admittedly this had been carried out between identical twins, whose immune systems did not recognize the incoming tissue as 'foreign'; but there were experimental suggestions that such a close relationship might not be necessary.

Immunosuppressive drug advances
In the early 1960s enormous strides were taken in kidney transplantation, and I avidly read

reports on the techniques being used to match tissues and reduce the risk of rejection. One way, still in use, is temporarily to suppress the action of the immune system by the use of so-called immunosuppressive drugs. However, by lowering the patient's immune guard the drugs lay him open to the risk of infections which can ride unchecked through the body, so that an organ may be successfully transplanted only for the patient to die from another disease altogether.

I realized that hazards such as these had to be faced and ultimately overcome if heart transplants were ever to become part and parcel of cardiac surgery. While I worked with my own investigations, others such as Norman Shumway and Denton Cooley, were joining the race to be first past the heart-transplant post.

In 1964 James D. Hardy, at the University of Mississippi, overcame the problem of donor

In 1958 Professor Vladimir Demikhov successfully transplanted a dog's heart into another dog during a four-hour operation at Leipzig University Clinic.

An X-ray of a cardiac catheter inserted into the heart.

availability by taking the heart from a chimpanzee and transplanting it into a 68-year-old man. The recipient did not survive for more than a few hours, the heart being too small for the task, but as an exercise in clinical procedure and human ambition Hardy's operation deserves the highest praise. Bit by bit, we were getting nearer to the day when one human's heart might be transplanted into another human's body, when one life might be extended by the most dramatic of all operations.

After my time at Minnesota I returned to South Africa, where I spent several years carrying out various surgical experiments alongside my regular work as a cardiac surgeon at the Groote Schuur Hospital in Cape Town. I repeated, for example, the dog-head graft, underlining to myself that surgical techniques were powerful enough to allow for greater things. However, my greatest concern was not connected with surgical techniques: I was much more worried about the fate of the transplanted heart once it was inside the recipient's body. As I wrote in a speech in 1963, 'The difficulty is how to maintain the existence of a foreign organ in a body without it being rejected. Yet even this will be overcome eventually . . .'

The first heart transplants

For four-and-a-half years I worked with my team at Groote Schuur to overcome this frustrating tendency of the immune system to oust grafted tissue. Like the US doctors Shumway and Lower we transplanted hearts from and into dogs, carrying out 48 such experimental operations with a high success rate. To get experience with immunosuppressive drugs we performed a kidney transplant in 1966 which worked perfectly, and acted as a dress rehearsal for a heart operation. This patient is still very much alive 20 years later. Her name is Mrs Black and at the time this caused much amusement in South Africa as her donor was a black man: headlines such as 'Mrs Black gets black kidney' were common. Spurred on by this operation, I was determined to put together all the knowledge we and others had accumulated on heart-surgery techniques, tissue compatibility and immunosuppressive drugs with the goal of achieving a heart transplant. This we did during

the night of 3 December 1967.

> Satisfied that the heart was finally free of air, I closed the hole in the pulmonary artery and released the clamp on the aorta. The heart became tense as blood rushed into the muscle – warm blood. This had an immediate and startling effect: the heart began to fibrillate. Where this movement had been a presage of death in Washkansky, it was here a sign of life – the first sign since its last beat in Denise Darvall three hours previously. The heart wanted to live – perhaps. Most certainly we wanted it to live, and our emotion was echoed in Ozzie's voice – consciously underplayed, yet betraying our hope.
>
> 'I'm getting some fibrillation and it looks . . . yes, it looks like it's becoming more active.'
>
> Perhaps it would start to beat on its own, and we waited for this to happen while the tension increased in the silent theatre. This was the peak we had struggled to find, climbing over two great barriers: co-ordinating the death of two hearts.
>
> (C. Barnard, *One Life*, Harrap, 1969.)

The heart of Denise Darvall had been transplanted into Louis Washkansky. This date was to become a milestone in cardiac surgery. Transplanting the heart had become feasible.

Washkansky and Blaiberg – the biggest steps

The recipient of the donated heart, Louis Washkansky, died 18 days later, the victim of both infection – the perennial bane of immunosuppression – and rejection. But it is an interesting reflection on the enthusiasm for heart-transplant surgery that had been building up at the time that, just three days later, a second transplant was carried out at the Maimonides Hospital in New York, this time on a baby. Again the recipient died shortly afterwards but when, the following January, I operated on the dentist Philip Blaiberg, he survived for 593 days, despite rejection problems. At the age of 58, he was, thanks to the operation, allowed a further year and a half of life, longer than he could otherwise have hoped for. When he was

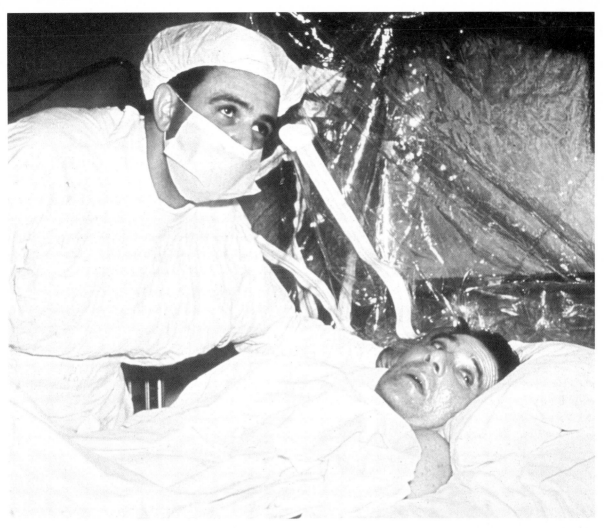

Louis Washkansky, the first human heart-transplant recipient, pictured after the operation.

interviewed after the operation, he was asked when he had first felt that the trauma had been worthwhile. He replied: 'As soon as I recovered from the anaesthetic and realized I could breathe properly again.'

Until that moment, I had not realized that I was developing a new personal philosophy towards the treatment of my patients. For me the goal of medicine is not the prolongation of life, it is improvement of the *quality* of life that is important. Living for a year unable to move without gasping for breath is one thing, living for a year like a normal person, walking, talking and even running, is quite another.

Philip Blaiberg, who survived for over a year-and-a-half after his transplant.

Survival times began to improve, but there were still some patients who succumbed very quickly as a result of infections, rejection or a failure in some other part of the body. Nowadays, 85 percent of recipients survive for at least one year, and many for much longer than this. These improvements in survival rates have come about as a result of three factors: improved diagnosis of rejection at an early stage; better anti-rejection drugs, such as Cyclosporin-A, which reduce the intensity, although not the frequency, of rejection; and improved methods of preserving donor organs, which have increased the chances of effective tissue-matching. Today, as a result of these advances, many patients are able to leave hospital after only three weeks.

SPARE PARTS FOR LIFE

A major difficulty in any transplant procedure is the shortage of 'spare' organs. It would be ideal if doctors could take the healthy organs of a dead person and store them in an organ bank, as blood can be stored in a blood bank. A centralized computer system could then ensure that organ and recipient were brought together wherever in the world they happened to be. But complex organs cannot be stored for more than about 48 hours. An American doctor, Gerald Klebanhoff, is reported to be developing a machine that might provide science-fiction-style suspended animation for whole bodies – even dead ones – for a day or two while suitable recipients are found. However, even this would not provide a wholly satisfactory spare-parts bank – even assuming enough donors could be found in the first place.

The real answer seems to lie in off-the-shelf parts, manufactured in their thousands in all shapes and sizes to fit into anybody in need of them. There would be no problems of availability beyond those of manufacturing or delivery delays and price. So far as the heart is concerned, the idea of artificial parts, and even a total replacement heart, has been around for some time. Over the years a variety of substances have been used for synthetic blood vessels: first Ivalon and then newer materials such as Teflon and Fluon, all of which can be cut to size and shape and will not decompose even after many years' wear as an artificial section of artery. Such substances have obviously become popular for making bypasses to clear blood vessel blockages – particularly since they are not easily rejected by the body.

As well as developing artificial blood vessels, however, medical scientists have developed replacement components for use in the heart. Initially surgeons were supplied with parts of parts; pieces of plastic, for instance, to replace faulty valve flaps. But in 1953 the brilliantly creative Dr. Charles A. Hufnagel, who had a taste for the emerging science of 'bioengineering' – the marriage of biological with manmade systems – inserted an industrial-type ball valve into the descending aorta to prevent back-flow. The early patients with this device in their chest would produce a distinct 'click' as the valve opened and closed but, progressively, the design was improved and, through the use of silicone balls, the unwanted noises were much reduced.

One of the first times an artificial heart powered by compressed air was used. Dr. Michael DeBakey is pictured here operating on a 65-year-old miner. At one stage the patient's own heart failed and the artificial heart took over until the patient's natural heart recovered.

In 1958, Hufnagel's coiled-spring valve was introduced; this had an anticipated life of 60 years – a remarkable achievement. Other valve designs include Albert Starr's 'Starr valve', which must still be opening and closing in many thousands of patients.

So the bioengineers, working alongside the cardiac surgeons, had given us replacement blood vessels, heart walls, even valves. How soon, though, would they be able to realize the ambition of a certain Dr. Kilb, who wrote in the *American Heart Journal* in May 1960, 'It is our aim to construct a pump that can permanently replace that irreparably sick human heart'?

Over the years a number of heart designs have been tested, particularly at the Division of Artificial Organs in Salt Lake City, where leading researchers, Robert Jarvik among them, are experimenting with machines that connect up to the body's pipework and provide a pumping action that comes close to the 'natural'.

Elsewhere in the USA, work is going on to develop a totally implantable heart powered by nuclear energy, using a tiny capsule of plutonium-238 to drive the mechanism as if it were a mini-reactor. As yet no human has been fitted with one of these because of the fear of radioactive contamination, but animals fitted with them have lived for some months.

How useful, to date, have artificial hearts been for human patients? Perhaps I can best answer that question by telling the story of a remarkable multiple operation which involved not only a synthetic organ but also a living transplant.

In the space of one phenomenal week, a young Dutch bus-driver, Willebrordus Meuffels, had no fewer than three different hearts keeping him alive. The first heart was his own, which after 36 years had become so diseased that a triple coronary-bypass operation was necessary. But, during the operation at the Texas Heart Institute, surgeons found that his flagging heart could not take the strain. A heart transplant was necessary to keep Meuffels alive. But where could they find a suitable donor?

A nationwide appeal was sent out, but meanwhile Meuffels had to have a means of pumping blood around his body. Enter Dr. Tetsuko Akutsu, bearing the answer in the form of an artificial heart which was made of plastic and powered by compressed air. The surgeons, led by the celebrated cardiac surgeon Dr. Denton Cooley, connected the artificial heart to the patient's circulation. Meuffels, semiconscious, lived on, while the heart of a young man who had died after a road crash was brought from Tennessee by air. Out came heart number two, and in its place went heart number three. The patient lived on for only a few days, being finally defeated by infection and other complications, but the point had been forcefully made that humans can accept artificial hearts as well as natural ones.

Today and the future

Long before any real-life Six Million Dollar Man has sprung into action, spare-part surgery, aided and abetted by improved transplantation techniques, has already evolved.

Since the mid-1950s, when I first embarked upon heart surgery, things have come a long way. In those days everything was difficult – even incisions to open the chest were made across rather than down the middle as they are now, making it hard to get access to the heart and its surroundings. Unlike today's heart surgeons, we had a lot of unfortunate losses; to carry out five open-heart operations in one week often meant losing five patients. Today success rates are much higher, and researchers are working on the ideal that artificial organs can be 'grown' in the laboratory: these will be neither completely natural nor wholly artificial, but a kind of tailor-made hybrid. The day will surely come when cardiac surgeons will be able to take off the shelf just the heart they require for a needy recipient, and carry out implantations with ease.

Meanwhile, back in the world of the present, each of us is possessed of an organ, the heart, with which we were born and which, just like all the other organs in the body, is prone to all manner of stresses, diseases, malfunctions and abnormalities. In the rest of *Your Healthy Heart* I shall be looking in detail at the heart's attackers, showing what can be done to counteract them and demonstrating how to avoid them altogether.

Dr. W. De Vries at Humana Hospital with an artificial heart ready for implantation.

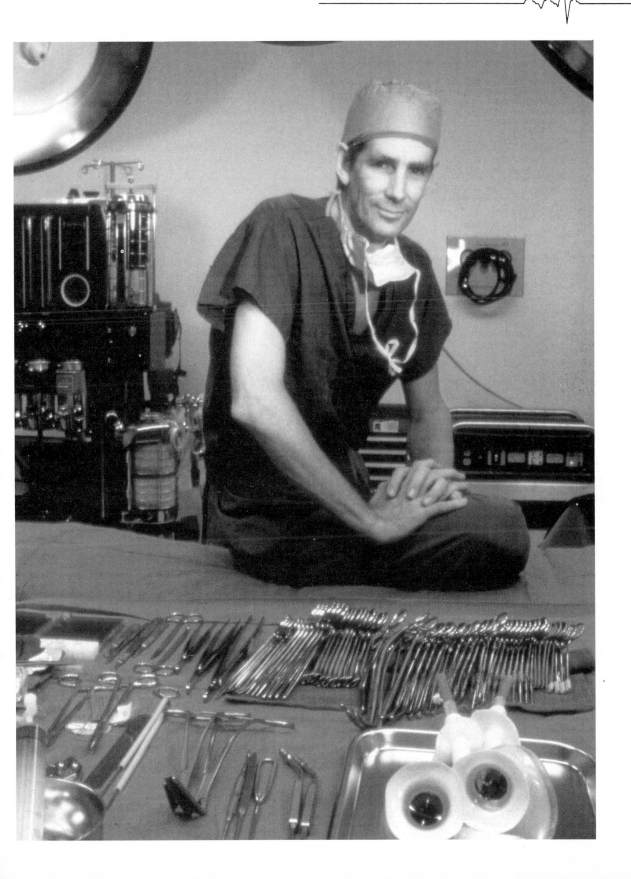

Chapter 2

Accidents of Birth:
congenital heart disorders

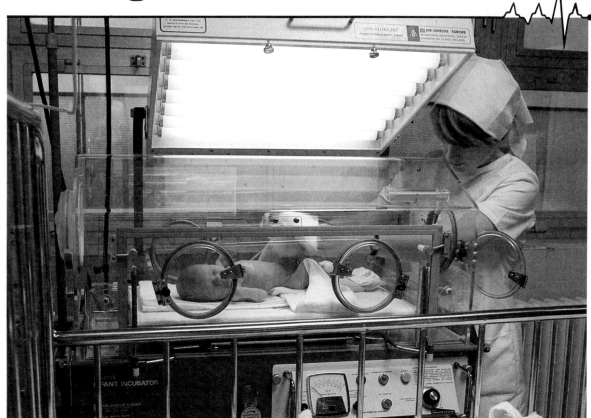

My teacher, Professor Charles Saint, made a point of considering six possible causes for any condition, be it a lump on the breast, a broken leg or a hole in the heart. These were: congenital, traumatic, inflammatory, neoplastic, ischemic, and unknown. For some reason, the heart is very prone to congenital disorders, whereas tumour (neoplastic) conditions are very rare. The high frequency of congenital malformations may perhaps be explained by the complex developmental processes the heart undergoes during the foetal stages, where a simple tube is transformed into the intricate three-dimensional, four-chambered structure so essential to life.

After an embryo has been forming in the womb for some days, the tiny foetal heart begins to beat, and blood ebbs and flows in circulation around the developing body. By the end of four weeks this flow is well established, and in a few more days the internal structures of the heart itself are near to their final shape, provided of course that all is well and that the baby in the womb has not, during these critical early weeks, developed abnormally in some way.

About one in every hundred babies is born with something wrong with its heart – a congenital disorder, brought about in the majority of cases by the mother-to-be catching an infection or suffering some other physiological

During pregnancy, the expectant mother should steer clear of drugs, smoking and alcohol.

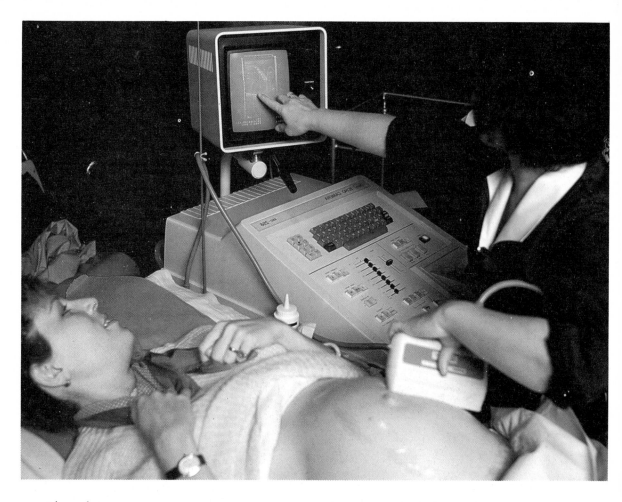

upset in early pregnancy.

Not all congenital disorders originate in this way. Some are inherited defects, carried on faulty genes passed down to the child from the parent or even, skipping a generation or two, from farther back in the family tree. These genetically determined heart conditions are very rare, so that a mother to whom a baby has been born with a congenital heart defect usually has only a very slim chance of producing a second child with the same disorder.

THE CAUSES OF CONGENITAL HEART DEFECTS

What are the reasons for these malformations? Metabolic disorders in the mother-to-be, such as diabetes or low thyroid-gland function (hypo-thyroidism) can cause heart malfunctions in offspring. Not that a diabetic woman should be

A pregnant mother is given a scan.

discouraged from becoming pregnant on the grounds that her condition will necessarily be injurious to her baby's heart – it need not be – but clearly the better controlled the condition the less the risk to the unborn child. Here the advice of your doctor, or genetic counsellor if you have access to one, is invaluable.

In addition, anything that reduces the oxygen content of the pregnant mother's blood can be dangerous, such as flying at high altitude in an unpressurized plane, or smoking.

Exposure to infections during pregnancy can be detrimental. It is firmly established that German measles (rubella), a common virus infection, can damage embryos. Sometimes the damage is so great that the embryo dies, but even children who survive may have a serious heart defect, among other complications. So it is better – if you can – to catch the disease a long time before becoming pregnant, and thus develop an immunity to it.

Less clear-cut is the relationship between other viral diseases (including familiar ailments such as influenza) and congenital heart disease. To be on the safe side, if you catch any infection at all during pregnancy report it to your doctor at once. You should also try to avoid exposing yourself to infection (especially, of course, rubella). But remember, even if a child is born with a heart defect, this may not necessarily be a serious one. Indeed, it may never produce any symptoms worth worrying about, let alone require treatment.

If possible, you should discuss vaccinations against such things as rubella with your doctor before you become pregnant.

No drugs, no alcohol, no cigarettes

Drugs taken for medical reasons can sometimes – although this is comparatively rare – damage the foetal heart and circulatory system. The best known example is that of thalidomide. Again, a full discussion with your doctor is needed if you are taking drugs regularly. It may be possible to switch from a potentially dangerous substance to something less harmful.

For a general set of guidelines you can do no better than follow the recommendation of the British Heart Foundation: 'During pregnancy at least, it is better to take no drugs whatsoever, even aspirin or so-called cold-cures, unless the doctor has recommended them.' And to this let me add another ban, at least for those critical

Hi-tech medicine. The ultrasound equipment at close quarters.

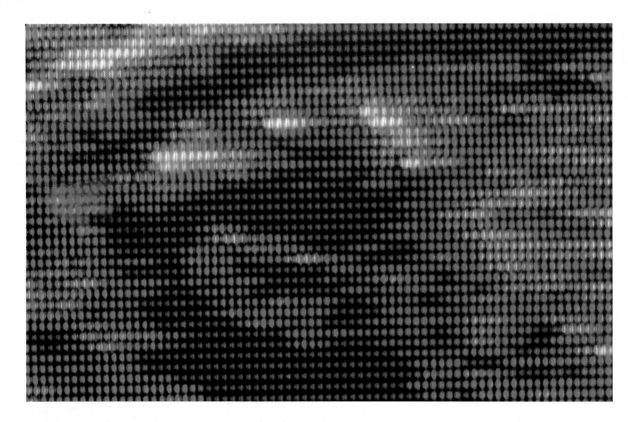

A close-up of a scan of the developing foetal heart.

early weeks of your pregnancy: no alcohol and no smoking. Heart disease or no heart disease, these two habits are unlikely to make for a healthy baby, and they may well do positive harm, even if you are fairly moderate in your intake.

CORRECTING CONGENITAL DEFECTS

It is here that heart surgeons are justified in blowing their own trumpets, because the prospects of a healthy life for a child born with one of the common congenital defects are nowadays extremely bright. If I look back over my own career, we seem to have gone from an attitude of 'no hope' for the baby with a malfunctioning heart to one of 'let's go'. Surgery has ensured that the great majority of children born with seriously defective hearts will live happy lives.

The diagnosticians, too, cannot be praised too highly – we no longer have to wait until a child is born before diagnosing a congenital heart defect. It is now possible to scan the heart of the baby in the womb, at no risk to mother or child, using

sound waves of very high frequency – ultrasound. This technique is often called echocardiography. At Guy's Hospital in London, techniques have been pioneered to spot heart defects at around 16 to 18 weeks after conception. Initially only major malformations, such as valve disorders or wrong connections to the heart, could be detected in this way, but now the ultrasonic scanner is being used for a wider

An echocardiograph of a normal foetal heart. Using this technique, defects can be detected before birth.

range of congenital problems.

If problems are detected, the parents have a choice: they may have the pregnancy terminated, or the mother can be taken to a specialist hospital with proper facilities for caring for the baby as soon as it is born.

Ultrasonic screening for congenital heart disease will almost certainly become a routine procedure. Not only will it help to provide early diagnosis but in some cases – for instance, that of arrhythmias in the foetus – it will enable doctors to treat their young patients before ever they see the light of day.

Helping the children

Parents of children with congenital heart defects often ask me, worried that too much rushing around will overtax their child, if they should impose restrictions on day-to-day movements. My answer is 'no'. Human beings – yes, children too – are very good at knowing when enough is enough, when their bodies are approaching their limits. Unless there is a very specific reason for certain activities to be proscribed – and your doctor has already spelled this out to you – do not worry unduly about a child swimming, skating, cycling and playing ball-games. Not only will the activity do no harm, it will prevent the young heart-sufferer from feeling different from everyone else, from being treated like a delicate flower, and from thinking of himself or herself as in any way 'special'.

If you are the parent of a child with a congenital heart defect, do not beat about the bush when your offspring asks questions. If a child suspects that something may be amiss, what with those visits to the hospital and those whispered consultations behind the screens, then your child's biggest enemy could be worry, and the best way of coping with it is to explain what is going on. Do not make the mistake of believing that having a heart defect somehow makes a child in any way insensitive or unintelligent. Relate the facts as you have understood them, or perhaps ask the heart consultant to help you out, and explain the need (if need there be) for an operation. However, if things are not going well, it is important that you don't allow your anxiety to show; children are very sensitive to mood.

From a physician's point of view, I have

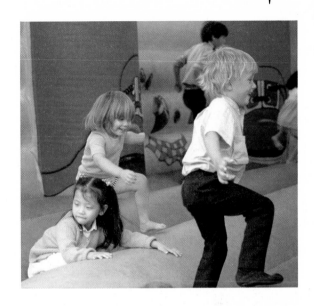

Children will normally regulate their own activity. They are very sensitive to being treated differently from others.

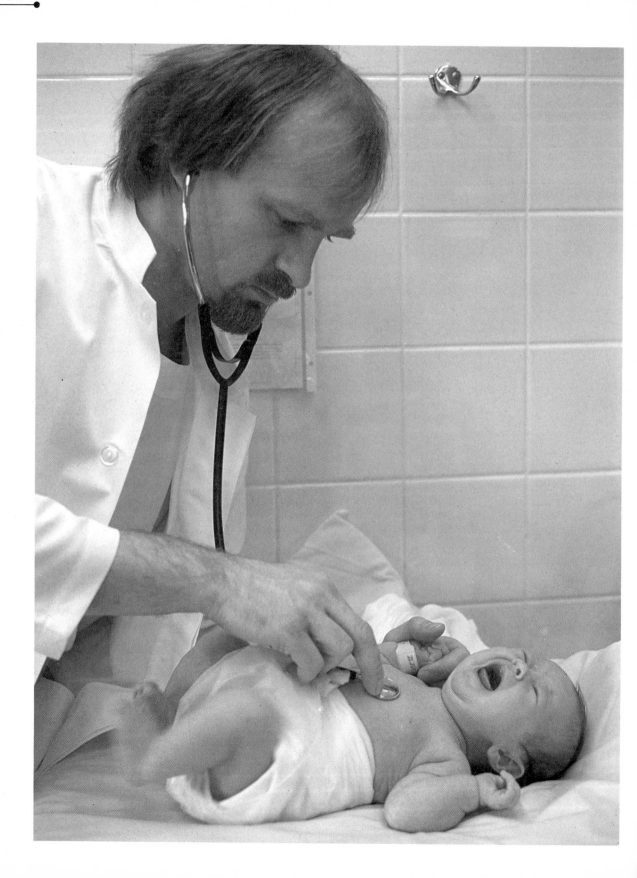

learned over the years that it is tragically easy to become emotionally involved with these young patients, so trusting and cheerful in adversity. But a surgeon must be objective, so I try to see the child only on the day before the operation.

While we are on the question of the child in hospital, I feel most strongly that there is no excuse for anything other than a total 'open door' policy. You should be allowed to see your child as much as possible – even staying with a youngster in the hospital if this is practicable – without any let or hindrance. I have performed hundreds of operations on all sorts of people, young and old, great and small, and I can tell you that it really matters to have the most important people in your life around in the post-op and recovery period. Not just to 'cheer up' the patient, but to give them the deep conviction that ultimately they matter, that their survival and fitness make the world a better place. Nothing quickens a child's will to recover and lead a normal life more than having the parents around, enjoying a bit of fun, sharing a family joke, reassuring and offering a constant reminder that you are looking forward to having him or her back with you soon. Ask any doctor about the will-to-live phenomenon and they will tell you that, without hope and the love of others, a person's recovery can be slowed down . . . and perhaps even stopped altogether.

HOLES IN THE HEART

The development of a baby's heart in the womb is a fascinating process. Quite early on it begins to form into its characteristic arrangement of four chambers, with the atria at the top and the ventricles at the bottom, each separated by walls or septa. These natural dividers develop progressively until, at birth, they form a proper blood-tight partition. Sometimes, however, the walls of these chambers fail to close properly. I have operated on a girl with hardly any septa at all: we had to use artificial materials to build substitute walls.

Usually, however, this underdevelopment is less severe, so that there is only a hole between

To stop children worrying, many hospitals now have pre-op familiarization sessions with young patients.

A doctor listens to the heartbeat of a new-born baby. In the West all babies are checked in detail for possible heart problems.

the two chambers. In the walls between the ventricles the holes may range in size from just a pinpoint up to a few millimetres or perhaps even a centimetre across. In the walls between the atria the hole sizes tend to be larger: between one and three centimetres. What are the medical hazards of these malformations?

Ventricular septal defects

Take first the effects of a hole between the ventricles. The resistance in the systemic circulation is normally higher than in the pulmonary circulation, so the pressure in the left ventricle is higher than that in the right. If there is a hole between the two, some already oxygenated blood will naturally, taking the line of least resistance, flow or 'shunt' from the left to the right ventricle, thereby overloading the right ventricle with blood, which it then has to pump through the lungs and return to the left-hand side

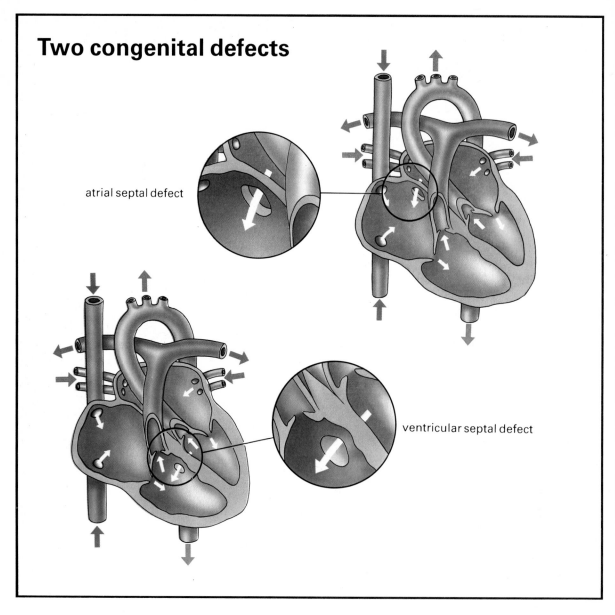

Two congenital defects

atrial septal defect

ventricular septal defect

of the heart. This means that the lungs become flooded, resulting in repeated chest infections.

One of the greatest dangers of this condition is that the increased amount of blood in the pulmonary circulation and the damage to the lungs may cause a gradual rise in the pulmonary resistance, until it reaches the point where it exceeds the systemic resistance. The shunt now reverses its direction – i.e., it goes from the right side of the heart to the left, so that unoxygenated blood is pumped into the arteries and around the body. This phenomenon, known

as Eisenmenger's Syndrome, is one of the ways in which a 'blue baby' can arise. This syndrome can occur also if the right and left sides of the heart are in communication for any other reason, for example, atrial septal defects and patent ductus, although this is less frequent. Until recently, these unfortunate patients could not be treated, but with the development of heart–lung transplants there is now some hope.

A tiny baby connected up to a heart–lung machine in readiness for open-heart surgery.

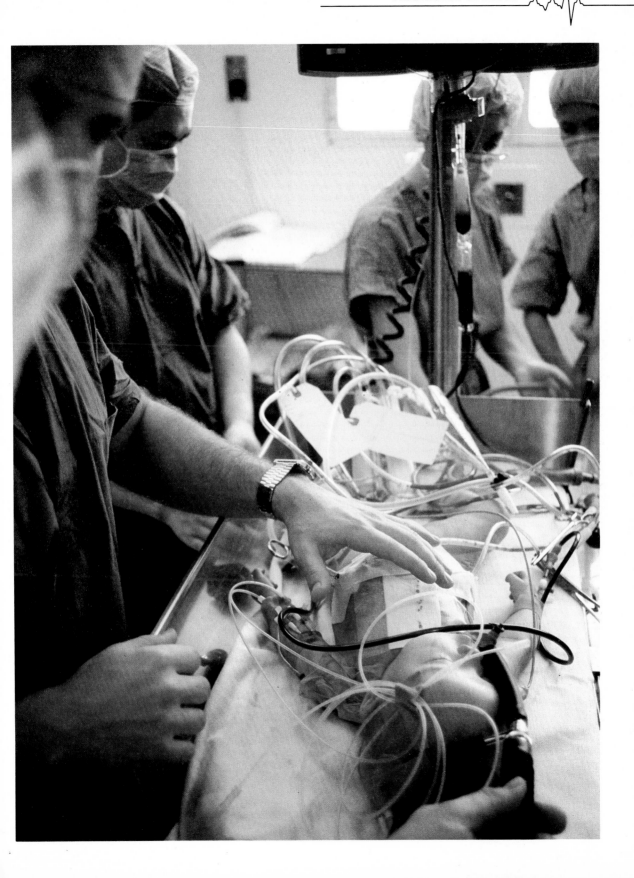

Atrial septal defects

Now think of a hole between the two atria, those two receiving chambers or 'marshalling yards' above the ventricles. As in the ventricles, the blood pressure on the left side is greater than that on the right, so that blood will pass through the hole from the left atrium into the right, and hence into the right ventricle and the pulmonary circulation, overfilling and overstressing both. The effects are not as damaging as with a ventricular opening; the symptoms come later and are less severe, but they are eventually debilitating, and may lead to heart failure, as with a ventricular septal defect.

Corrective surgery

If it is decided to go ahead with surgery, this should only be attempted using a total bypass of the whole cardiopulmonary system. In other words the heart–lung machine must take over the work of the heart long enough for the hole to be closed.

Make no mistake about my position on any form of surgery to the heart. It may be technically feasible and scientifically clever to perform these feats, but the patient must come first. The mere fact that a hole can be closed using open-heart procedures does not of itself warrant their use. The long- and short-term risks and benefits have to be weighed up cautiously. Indeed, some ventricular septal defects are so small that they do not affect the patient's health, and sometimes they actually close themselves spontaneously; usually this takes place in the first year or two of life.

Holes in the heart can be closed in two ways. Either the edges can be pulled together and sutured directly or one can use a 'patch' of plastic material or of the body's own tissue, such as a piece of pericardium (the tissue surrounding the heart). In the past we used to correct ventricular septal defects by cutting into the right ventricles, but this is not very desirable, especially when the right ventricle is already under abnormal pressure. Today, unless the septal defect is in a very awkward place, we repair it by cutting into the right atrium and approaching the ventricular septum through the tricuspid valve.

When to operate? Because of the high risk of the shunt's direction reversing, treatment is

a

urgent. If the shunt does reverse the defect becomes inoperable because, once the shunt is from right to left, the hole in the septum acts as a safety valve, relieving the pressure in the right ventricle. If the aperture is closed the patient will go into severe right-heart failure and die.

Not so long ago, when it was very risky to operate on the hearts of very young children, a stop-gap operation was carried out. A plastic band was put around the pulmonary artery to narrow it so the resistance in the pulmonary circuit was increased (although it still remained lower than in the systemic circulation), and thereby the rate of the initial left-to-right shunt was reduced. This meant that the lungs did not become flooded to such an extent that pulmonary resistance became higher than the systemic resistance, and so a reversal in the direction of the shunt was avoided. Today, now that we can operate on babies only a few hours old and weighing only 1-1.5 kg, this interim procedure has been virtually abandoned.

The procedures for atrial-septal-defect operations are very similar. However, because the atrial septum is thinner than the ventricular septum, it is usually sutured directly, rather than patched. Because there is little danger of

a)   X-ray of mitral valve disease.
b)   X-ray of aortic stenosis.
c)   X-ray of Tetralogy of Fallot.

b

c

shunt-reversal with atrial septal defects, correction is usually delayed until the child is bigger and stronger. The symptoms of these defects are relatively benign, so it is more important that operations are carried out only when the surgical team have the skill to guarantee virtually 100 percent success. Properly performed, however, closures of atrial septal defects are spectacularly effective, and deaths uncommon.

CONGENITAL OBSTRUCTIONS TO THE FREE-FLOW OF BLOOD

There are three causes of congenital obstructions; these can often be serious, and must be corrected urgently. They are:

1   Stenosed valves due to fusion of the cusps, especially in the pulmonary valve but also in the aortic and tricuspid valves. Congenital stenosis of the mitral valve is rare.

2   Underdevelopment of an area due to decreased flow of blood to the heart. This can be a major problem in the Tetralogy of Fallot (see below).

3   Overgrowth of muscle tissue in the heart.

The correction of these conditions is often a complex procedure, involving the opening of the valves (which can be very tricky with the aortic valve, as any backflow can be fatal); enlarging underdeveloped areas with grafts from the patient's own tissues or with artificial materials such as Teflon, or even bypassing the area if it is very underdeveloped; and, in the event of an overgrowth, cutting away obstructing muscle bands. Techniques are improving all the time.

THE TETRALOGY OF FALLOT AND PULMONARY STENOSIS

Another condition which can cause cyanotic congenital heart disease (as the 'blue baby' syndrome is technically known) is the Tetralogy of Fallot. This condition, which derives its name from Étienne-Louis-Arthur Fallot, who first described it in 1880, is for some reason much more common in boys than in girls. Here again

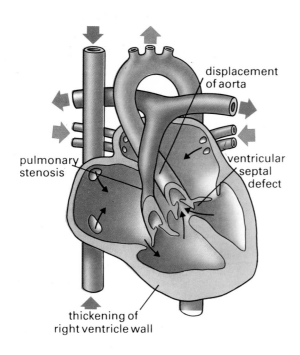

displacement
of aorta

pulmonary
stenosis

ventricular
septal
defect

thickening of
right ventricle wall

Tetralogy of Fallot

the blueness is due to the reversal of a shunt between the right and left ventricles, causing deoxygenated blood to circulate. This reversal is not, however, caused by changes in the pulmonary system's resistance but is due to the resistance posed by the narrowing and obstruction of the outflow of the right ventricle. Dr. Fallot thought that there were four congenital defects involved, hence the term 'Tetralogy':

1 An opening between the ventricles – a ventricular septal defect.

2 A blocked or stenosed pulmonary valve.

3 An aorta that emerges from both ventricles instead of just the left ventricle.

4 An enlargement of the right ventricle.

In fact, the second two defects develop later as a result of the ventricular septal defect and the pulmonary valve defect. If these latter conditions

are treated, the enlargement of the right ventricle and the distortion of the position of the aorta rectify themselves.

The severity of the condition, which will determine the symptoms of the patient and the degree of cyanosis (blueness), is itself determined by the degree of the obstruction to the outflow from the right ventricle to the lungs caused by one or a combination of the reasons mentioned in this context earlier. If the obstruction is mild, little or no blueness will show – this is known as 'acyanotic tetralogy'. If the obstruction is severe, however, the child will be very incapacitated: without treatment, such infants are prone to convulsions and bouts of unconsciousness during feeding or crying, their growth is impaired, and the expected milestones of normal development are delayed. Moreover, these children are susceptible to infections, such as bacterial endocarditis. Yet another complication is that, because the blood is inadequately oxygenated, it tries to make up for its own deficiency by manufacturing more than its usual quantity of red cells; as a result, it becomes very thick and viscous, and this in turn can lead to problems with blocked arteries and veins, especially in the brain.

Left to itself, the Tetralogy of Fallot is a desperately unkind condition. Without drastic treatment, nine out of ten 'blue babies' would die before the age of twenty-five, having struggled through years of considerable disability and discomfort. So the arguments are very much in favour of surgery, despite the risks attendant on any operation of this magnitude.

Correcting the Tetralogy of Fallot
Correcting the condition basically involves first closing the ventricular septal defect (as described) and then relieving the obstruction to the outflow of the right ventricle. In very severe cases, relieving the obstruction may entail cutting out any overgrowth of muscle, opening up the narrowed valve, and enlarging the underdeveloped area with a gusset.

At what age should a complete correction be performed? Assuming that there is adequate development of the right ventricular outflow tract and pulmonary arteries, a complete correction can be done at any age. If there is inadequate development and reconstruction is needed, then the child is tided over by use of a palliative procedure until the age of two to three years. There are various palliative procedures, but all are designed to increase blood-flow to the lungs and thereby improve oxygenation. One way is to create a shunt between a systemic artery and the pulmonary artery; another is partially to relieve the obstruction to the right ventricular outflow by, for example, pulmonary valvotomy (improving the functioning of the pulmonary valve).

Correcting the Tetralogy of Fallot is one of the most rewarding operations a surgeon can do. A sickly, blue child is transformed within a matter of hours into a healthy, pink, lively individual. The effect seems miraculous.

The surgical correction of the Tetralogy of Fallot.

OTHER CORRECTIVE SURGERY

So far I have talked about shunts between the pulmonary and aortic circulations and obstructions inside the heart. Shunts and obstructions can occur also outside the heart, such as the shunt caused by the ductus arteriosis not closing properly after birth (patent ductus arteriosus). This causes a left-to-right shunt, and the aperture needs to be closed or the same dangerous consequences as with ventricular septal defects can occur. The operation for patent ductus is simpler than that for septal defects: there is no need for a heart–lung machine or open-heart surgery. The chest is opened and the duct is either tied off (less popular as the condition can sometimes recur) or clamped, severed and sewn. This operation is done today with great success and hardly any

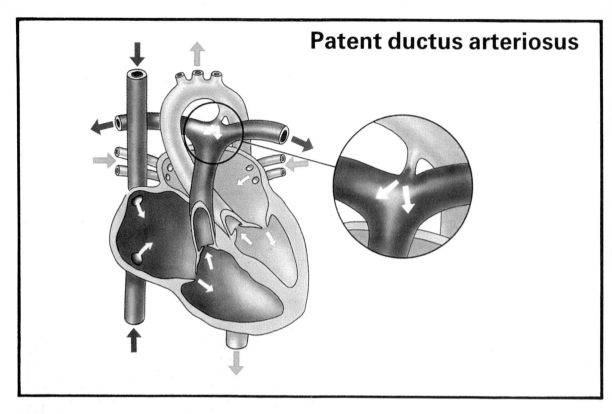

Patent ductus arteriosus

mortality. In the old days, however, the operation took nearly all day and it was very dangerous – I remember one child coming out of theatre with two clamps still in her chest because we just couldn't control the bleeding. This kind of drama rarely happens in modern heart surgery.

An example of an obstruction to the free flow of blood that occurs outside the heart is coarctation of the aorta. This is a narrowing in the descending aorta at just about the place where the patent ductus has closed and could be a result of over-closure of the ductus, although we are still not quite sure. The correction of this condition is similar to that for a narrowing inside the heart, but a heart–lung machine does not have to be used. The most common method is to control the flow in the aorta using clamps above and below the obstruction, and then to slit open the artery and put a patch on it to enlarge it. There is also a new technique which uses a flap from the subclavian artery as a patch.

I have had a great deal of success with resection of the narrowed area, joining the cut ends by direct anastomosis. On rare occasions, if the gap is too big, a small graft may be needed.

MULTIPLE PROBLEMS, MULTIPLE SOLUTIONS

A child may well be born with two or more malfunctions in his or her cardiac system – for example, patent ductus *and* a ventricular septal defect. In such cases all the considerations I have mentioned concerning the timing, procedures and complications of an operation are made more complex. Offsetting this, however, are the undeniably spectacular advances in the surgical treatment of all the congenital disorders; by 'treatment' I mean not just a suturing method here or a plastic insert there, but the whole understanding of the nature of these hitherto insoluble problems, such as pulmonary atresia, tricuspidatresia, and transposition of the aorta and the pulmonary artery. Details of these and other less common conditions can be found in the specialist literature.

Nine congenital defects
I can best illustrate these dramatic advances by telling you about an operation carried out in 1982 at the world-famous Great Ormond Street

Hospital for Sick Children, London. The patient was a West German boy, 13-year-old Frank Weyrauch, who came to the attention of doctors with no fewer than nine – yes, *nine* – congenital defects. The most serious was the complete absence of a dividing septum between the two atria, so that both pumps were effectively fused into one; in addition, instead of a pair of non-return valves feeding into the ventricles, he had only one. On top of these gross defects were seven other malformations. Without surgery Frank would have been condemned to a very short life. What is more, until quite recently, even if surgery had been attempted it would have taken the form of a series of major operations, each designed to correct one fault at a time.

However, under the direction of Jaroslav Stark, a team of surgeons tackled Frank's problems in just one mega-operation. They took existing body-tissues to form a wall across the two atria, then created an extra one-way valve to provide another outlet into the ventricles. After that they closed a ventricular septal defect and worked on an abnormal arrangement of major blood vessels leading to and from the heart. In other words, they performed in one operation virtually everything I have been describing in the whole of this chapter, demonstrating conclusively that, with the will, the funds and the necessary technology, surgery for correcting congenital heart defects ranks, in terms of success, in the very top league. Almost anything seems possible.

An historic occasion. In 1961 the Italian surgeon Achille Dogliotti completed an amazing operation, in which he transferred the heart of a four-year-old boy from the right to the left side of his body.

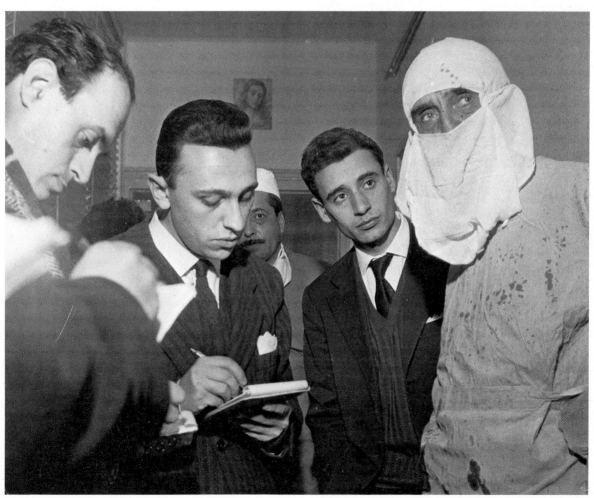

Chapter 3
Acquired Heart Disease:
diagnosing the dangers

I am not superstitious. I do not subscribe to the view that we poor mortals are the playthings of the gods and their paranormal powers; that all our lives are manipulated like some grand puppet show.

Yet I do most firmly believe in the idea of good and bad luck in the sense of statistical risk. Of all the millions of healthy babies born into the world each year, a certain unlucky percentage will carry in their genes – those biochemical bearers of coded messages that dictate what we are – the information that spells disease and illness. It may be that the condition manifests itself immediately, as with some congenital heart defects, or it may emerge later in life thanks to a cruel delayed action on the part of the aberrant genes which, while a person has been showing no symptoms at all, have all the while been ensuring his or her ultimate vulnerability.

Eventually, and this really is an exciting prospect, it may become possible not only to predict genetic disorders of all kinds but even perhaps to correct them by tinkering with the make-up of the genes themselves, thereby 'engineering' good health. But for the present we have to accept the hand we are dealt.

That said, however, so far as heart disease is concerned, the risks of succumbing are not at all beyond our control. If we set aside congenital disorders and look at the overwhelming majority of 'heart conditions' in general, we find that these are not imposed upon us willy-nilly but acquired as a result of our lifestyle. The hands that pull the strings are yours and mine.

Far and away the most common and most devastating form of heart disease in developed countries is coronary heart disease – CHD, initials that we might use also to spell out this message I shall be putting across throughout the rest of this book: *Care Helps Deter*. Coronary heart disease is undeniably the great scourge of modern, affluent, well-fed society (just as infections such as tuberculosis scythed down our ancestors who lived in less sanitary times). If CHD has increased in statistical frequency as our lifestyle has changed, then it stands to reason that there are things about the modern world that contribute towards its spread. If we understand these factors and try to modify our way of living accordingly, we ought to be able to reduce the risks. CHD: Care Helps Deter.

CORONARY HEART DISEASE: A CIVILIZED COMPLAINT

Coronary heart disease – the outcome of a restricted or even blocked supply of blood to the heart muscle itself – is by no means a new phenomenon. We know this from historical records which show that its most dramatic manifestation, sudden death from a heart attack (the much-feared 'coronary' that strikes the middle-aged male so frequently), stretches way back to antiquity. There is, for instance, the case on record of a certain Roman senator who, having delivered to the Senate a powerful speech, collapsed and expired on leaving the debating hall.

- damaged endothelium (vessel lining)

FATTY STREAK lipid-filled smooth muscle cell

FIBROUS PLAQUE collagen and elastic fibres
- lipids

- thrombus
- haemorrhage
- lipids

Hardening of the arteries. The process begins with damage to the lining of the blood vessel: the smooth muscle cells then increase and lipid (fatty) streaks accumulate. Collagen and elastic fibres develop, forming a fibrous plaque which protrudes into the blood vessel. Further tissue destruction and calcification with haemorrhage is the final advanced stage.

Atherosclerosis

This is the degeneration of the inner artery lining, caused by the build-up of fatty substances – as distinct from arteriosclerosis, which is the overall medical term for 'hardening of the arteries'. The internal wall of a healthy artery is smooth and elastic, enabling blood to flow freely through on its way to the body's organs from the heart. Atherosclerosis develops when fatty streaks start to form inside the artery, often at stress points where branching occurs or where the wall is already damaged. The deposits thicken, forming atheroma, hard masses of fatty tissue that erode the wall and further narrow the arterial pathway, thus impairing the flow of blood. Atheroma builds up to form harder masses called plaque; the process is made worse by platelets, the blood's clotting elements, getting trapped on the plaque.

Atherosclerosis is usually symptomless until it becomes well advanced, when a body organ supplied by damaged or blocked arteries begins to suffer from lack of blood, and therefore lack of oxygen.

For example blockages in the arteries supplying the brain can lead to cerebral haemorrhage, or stroke; if the heart's own supply arteries are blocked, coronary artery disease will develop. Sometimes heart pain – angina – results from the stress put on severely narrowed coronary arteries. A heart attack occurs when the blood supplying the heart muscle is suddenly and severely reduced by a clot of blood – a thrombosis – lodged in a coronary artery.

A vast number of people in advanced industrial societies have some degree of atherosclerosis; it is known to start early in life, usually reaching an advanced stage around or beyond middle age. A high level of blood cholesterol seems to contribute towards the condition, so that although the regulation of blood cholesterol is still not fully understood, it is safe to say that you can reduce the chance of developing atherosclerosis by minimizing your overall fat intake, particularly animal fats. Smoking and obesity also lead to greater susceptibility.

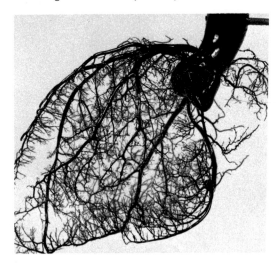

A cast of normal coronary arteries in a sixteen-year-old (above).

A cast of coronary arteries damaged by atherosclerosis.

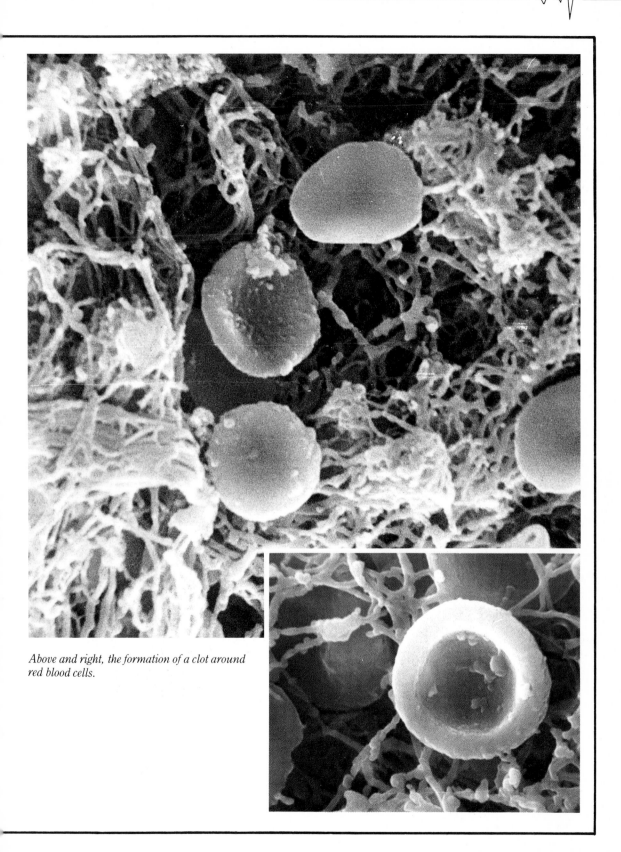

Above and right, the formation of a clot around red blood cells.

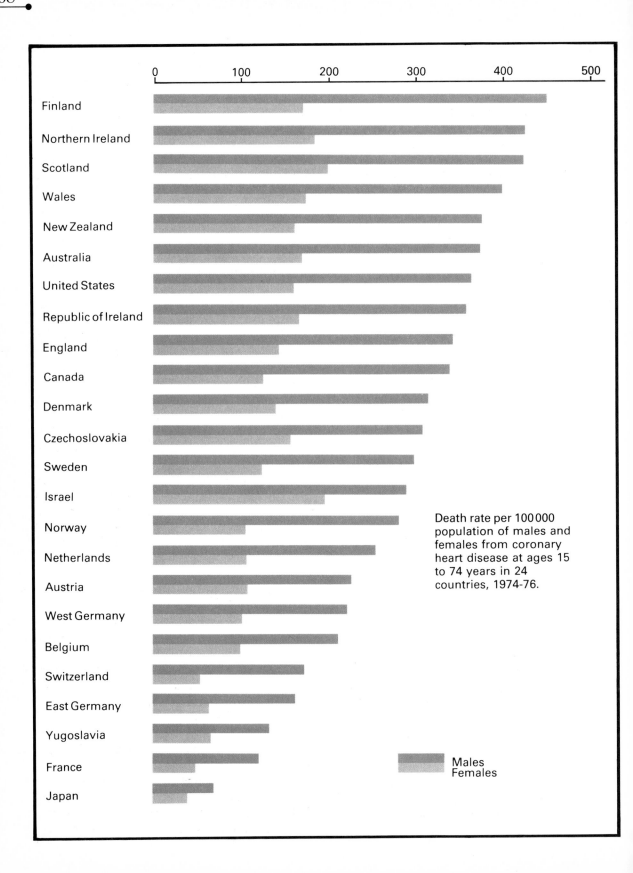

Death rate per 100 000 population of males and females from coronary heart disease at ages 15 to 74 years in 24 countries, 1974-76.

Males
Females

Nevertheless, the menace of coronary heart disease appears to be growing in step with the spread of urbanized, industrialized, affluent society. When the celebrated Sir William Osler, a medical pioneer at the Johns Hopkins Medical School in the USA, delivered a classic series of lectures in London in 1910, he could point to only a few cases of coronary heart disease that he had encountered in his long career. Today the charts tell their own story. Coronary heart disease, in the space of a few short decades, has streaked ahead to become the league leader in the West as a cause of death among middle-aged men.

Stark facts

Do not let any distrust of statistics fog your perceptions of the problem of CHD. Here are some sober facts about the situation in Western Europe and the USA:

CHD is on the increase most markedly among younger people, in the 35 to 44 age-group. In fact, in England and Wales the death-rate in this age-group doubled in just 15 years, from 1950 to 1965.

Men are decidedly more at risk than women but – and this is significant – the female side of the population is catching up. In England after 1960 the graph of female deaths from CHD has been sharply on the upturn.

Of every 1000 men now aged 40, 200 will suffer at least one heart attack before they reach 65.

Comparing the figures from different countries shows some interesting features that we can use to identify where the CHD risks come from. In the USA the overall death-rate from CHD shot up by 50 percent between 1940 and 1960, that great boom period in the 'American way of life' when people, to appropriate Harold Macmillan's phrase, 'never had it so good'. Look too at Finland, and, close behind in the unenviable position of runners-up, Northern Ireland and Scotland. These nations are at the very top of the

The incidence of CHD varies dramatically from country to country, clearly demonstrating the link between CHD and lifestyle.

coronary-mortality league – while Japan nestles comfortably at the very bottom.

What is the difference? You might be tempted to argue that the Japanese have some inbuilt, racially determined advantage over those living in the West, some factor that makes them by nature less prone to succumb. But then you have to revise that opinion when you learn that CHD-rates among Japanese who emigrate to the USA and live there for some years do not remain low, but instead fall into line with those of the host nation.

The good news is that in the USA things do seem to be improving. Recent figures from the World Health Organization show that in the last few years the US death-rates have begun to decline – by as much as 27 percent between 1968 and 1976. Why has this happened? A freak of the figures? An accident of fate? Or could it be that Americans have begun to change their lifestyle in ways that might make an impact on the prevalence of the arch enemy?

Finally, is it any coincidence that CHD, for all its ravages in the industrialized world, is uncommon in the Third World? Indeed, the less contact there is with 'civilization' the fewer CHD cases seem to be recorded.

Note, however, that statistics can be misleading. Better diagnostic techniques must explain at least some of the recorded increase in the incidence of CHD, and improved treatment at least some of the reduction in the death-rate.

DIAGNOSING HEART DISEASE: THE SYMPTOMS

There is an old proverb that runs 'Every man is a fool or a physician', the implication being that anybody who does not know enough about health and medical matters to act as his own doctor must be a fool. After all, we are tuned into our own bodies and their vagaries in a unique way. For instance, for years now I have suffered from a painful type of arthritis which affects mostly the joints of my hands and feet. When I wake up in the morning I *know* whether it is going to be a good or a bad day. It is as if my brain were tuned to exactly the right frequency to receive faint tell-tale signals from my body that indicate how my joints will respond to the day ahead. That kind of knowledge becomes the starting point for any diagnosis of illness.

That said, do not let us take the self-healing notion too far. If there is any possibility that you are suffering from heart disease you cannot go it alone. You need your doctor, not just to provide help in treating the condition, but to help you to identify it. I stress that after long years of meeting doctors who tell me time after time that most people who come to them saying, 'I think it's my heart, Doctor', have made a mis-diagnosis. Heart disease can be confused with other conditions which have practically identical signs and symptoms that the untrained eye can misinterpret. That said, if you have the slightest suspicion, consult your doctor – particularly since some of these conditions can be quite serious in themselves.

Chest pain

One of the most common and typical indicators of CHD is pain in the chest. In its chronic form, chest pain – *angina pectoris* – is usually activated by exertion, emotional reactions, a heavy meal or exposure to cold. It will often disappear after a few minutes' rest but, if severe, may persist for 30 minutes or more.

The pain is very characteristic. It is like a gripping, vice-like feeling of pressure behind the breastbone which can radiate to the left shoulder and arm and continue to the right arm, too. The neck and jaw may also feel the burning pressure, the 'heaviness' of an ache that, once subsided, leaves you with a deep feeling of relief. Usually only rest will make angina subside, although a few people whose pain is brought on through exercise are known to be able to 'walk through pain' – that is, they continue their activity until they experience relief.

That is the true angina, the sign that coronary heart disease is the problem. But we get all manner of chest pains – in fact, a total of 101 different causes of chest pain have been identified, so there is no need to equate 'pain in the chest' with 'heart disease' straight away. Here are some false trails.

Left chest pain A dull ache, sometimes with momentary sharp stabs of pain roughly where the heart is located. This type of pain is, unlike

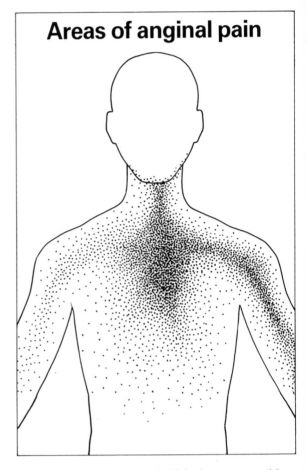

Areas of anginal pain

Anginal pain is most frequently felt in the upper part of the chest, neck and jaw, but will often extend to the left shoulder and arm. In severe angina, the right side of the body is also affected.

angina, not dependent on physical exertion and may last for some hours at a time. The cause could be nervous in origin, possibly made worse by the very act of worrying about having a heart condition!

Brief stabbing pains Again unrelated to exertion, these pains are often caused by air being trapped under the diaphragm – 'wind' you might call it. The cause is over-rapid eating, so that excess air is swallowed in the process. Indigestion and angina can cause very similar symptoms. A friend of mine, Professor James Lowe, woke up one night and went to get some milk to calm his 'indigestion', but it was actually angina he was suffering from. Even the experts can be fooled without a proper physical examination.

Activity-related pain   Unusually heavy physical stresses may strain the chest cage and spine, causing a persistent pain in the centre of the chest. The pain is due to damage to the joints in the ribs or, if not, to some muscle other than the heart. Severe rib pains caused by a pinched nerve are also sometimes mistaken for CHD symptom. The pain may persist for several days but responds to treatment designed to reduce inflamed muscles and nerve fibres.

To sum up, angina pain is not the same as other types of chest pain. If you have any discomfort in the chest area do two things: see your doctor, and do not make up your mind about what is wrong with you until you have been examined.

Breathlessness

Another key symptom is breathlessness. When the heart is starting to fail, a person gets increasingly out of breath after physical exertion. He or she may become breathless even when just lying down. Together with shortness of breath, the sufferer may also suffer tiredness and listlessness, with coldness in the limbs.

Many people feel breathless as they get older, finding themselves seemingly unable to draw a deep full breath of air into their lungs, but this is not the same as the breathlessness experienced by people in the early stages of heart failure who are over-exerting themselves. Moreover, there are many other conditions that will cause this symptom, among them bronchitis, asthma, dietary deficiencies, emphysema, pneumonia, obesity, lung cancer, cystic fibrosis and so on. So, as a symptom, breathlessness is always to be taken seriously, but not always to be thought of as necessarily indicative of heart disease.

Heartbeat

The same is true of abnormal heartbeat, especially palpitations – a stronger or faster than normal beat does not necessarily spell trouble. If you are out of condition and run upstairs rapidly, your heart may continue pounding quickly for some time after you have stopped running. If you are suffering from stress of are worried a similar

effect may be felt. But rarely is this due to some fundamental disorder of heart rhythm.

The classic proof of this is the so-called 'soldier's heart' noticed during the First World War and later during the Second, when it was dubbed 'effort syndrome'. Newly recruited soldiers in intensive training will often get a rapid 100-beats-to-a-minute pounding of the heart, together with a dull pain in the chest on the left side. The signs seem to point to heart disease, but on closer inspection it appears that the people thus affected often lose their symptoms with further training.

Fainting

Many people fear, too, that fainting attacks herald heart disease. Again the evidence is to the contrary. It is true that certain severe heart disorders – such as heart failure due to shock, obstruction of the aortic valve and heart-beat aberrations – will result in a temporary failure of blood-supply to the brain and hence in fainting, but this occurs only in the minority of cases. Fainting is a very common symptom of medical malfunctioning, and as likely as not is quite unconnected with the heart's competence.

Angina pectoris is really only a symptom of CHD. For other types of heart disease, one can usefully divide the symptoms of heart disease up into right heart failure, which causes congestion of the body and shows up in odoema of the feet, especially during the day. At night one finds that, because the patient is lying flat, oedema may develop over the sacrum. There may also be enlargement of the liver, which can result in the patient complaining of pain in this area. Sometimes the neck veins become distended and there can be congestion of the kidney.

Left-sided failure causes congestion of the lungs and the symptoms the patient presents with are shortness of breath, at first only during exercise but then at rest as well. Very characteristic is a type of breathlessness which we call cardiac asthma or *paraxysmal nocturnal dyspnoea*, where the patient suddenly wakes up at night short of breath; interestingly, when the patient sits up the breathlessness usually disappears. Of course, one of the main symptoms of wet and congested lungs is coughing and this cough may produce phlegm. If both the left and the right sides of the heart are failing the symptoms can appear in many different combinations.

DIAGNOSTIC TOOLS OF THE TRADE

The signs of heart disease can be misleading, even wildly so – but if you have any of the above symptoms it is only by taking things a stage further and visiting your physician that a positive or negative diagnosis can be made. You should not hesitate to arrange that visit, and you should report any symptoms that recur or cause you to feel concern.

Soldiers training. New recruits can develop a rapidly pounding heart and a dull pain – the symptoms go after further training.

Hear! Hear!

Laënnec's Stethoscope

Modern physicians first place their stethoscopes over areas of the chest most likely to yield abnormal sounds associated with the four cardiac valves.

Nothing identifies a doctor so readily as the stethoscope. It is the unmistakable tool of his trade, without which he would not seem fully or even partially equipped. But in fact the use of an instrument for listening to sounds in the chest *(stethos)* did not emerge until the beginning of the nineteenth century. Up until then, physicians had followed the example of the ancient Greek, Hippocrates, and listened to the sounds of the heart and lungs by placing an ear close to the chest – 'immediate auscultation', as it is called.

Then in 1816 René Laënnec invented an instrument for mediate auscultation – listening with an intervening device – which revolutionized the whole procedure of diagnosing heart disorders. Initially he used a rolled tube of paper, later a hollow wooden cylinder. Although different in outward form from the modern instrument, with its flexible tubing and double earpiece, Laënnec's device was basically the same as is used today. Indeed, the original, straight stethoscope is still used for certain tasks such as listening to the heart of the unborn baby.

However, the stethoscope in itself is not enough. To use it properly for diagnostic purposes requires clinical skill and knowledge.

Let us imagine, then, that you have decided to seek expert help. How does a doctor set about making a diagnosis, and how might he decide that the cause of the problem is indeed a faulty heart or circulatory system?

It is important that the process begins with your medical history: you must give your doctor a detailed account of symptoms (type, how long, severity, peculiarities, etc.) and any indication of a family tendency towards various illnesses. A detailed description at this stage can often give the skilful doctor an insight into the true nature of your condition even before he turns to a full physical examination.

External examination

During the initial physical examination the doctor attempts to follow up and confirm any hunches he may have had, at the same time retaining an open mind about the cause of the patient's distress. It is surprising to the lay person to learn how much can be inferred by the physician from this basic external examination. The doctor will first use his senses of sight and touch to search for distended neck veins, swelling in the legs or at the base of the spine and for any abnormal veins that one can see over the stomach. The doctor will 'palpate' the heart so that he can feel the beat – for example, if there is a strong apex beat, this

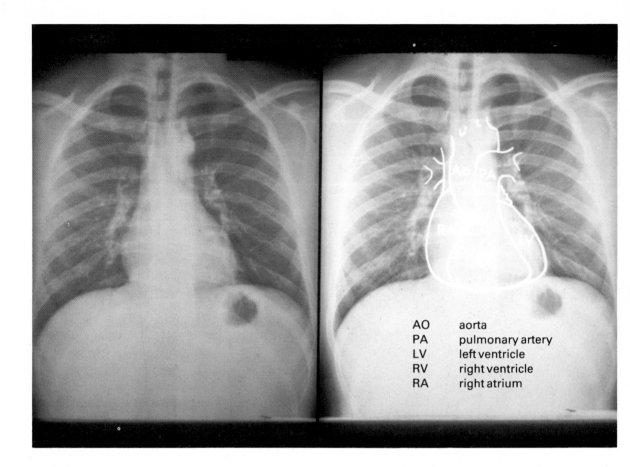

AO	aorta
PA	pulmonary artery
LV	left ventricle
RV	right ventricle
RA	right atrium

is indicative of an enlarged left ventricle. The doctor can actually feel abnormal sounds and murmurs. The next step is auscultation, where the stethoscope is used to hear more precisely what goes on in the heart in order to detect the characteristic murmurs as the blood flows through malfunctioning heart valves.

As a matter of fact, heart murmurs – extra sounds over and above the regular heartbeat – are much more common than you might think. Often new-born babies have them, although most disappear spontaneously. And not all murmurs indicate heart disease. Many adults have extraneous murmurs, called innocent murmurs, which do not appear to affect the function of the heart at all.

X-rays

After the physical examination the patient may be given a straight X-ray. This will show up enlarged chambers and abnormal beats. The interpretation of X-rays is a highly specialized job.

A simple X-ray of the chest can tell the skilled physician much about the condition of the heart. On the right, the same X-ray is shown with the main blood vessels and chambers identified.

The electrocardiograph

In many cases the family doctor will want a second opinion from a cardiologist, who has the added advantage of being able to draw on a wider range of medical technology. One of the most frequently used tools of the cardiologist's trade is the electrocardiograph – the ECG, sometimes known in the USA as the EKG. The ECG is in fact a highly sensitive galvanometer, an instrument which measures differences in electrical potential. Coupled to the galvanometer is a time-marker and a recorder.

When the heart beats, there are minute changes in the electrical currents transmitted through the heart muscle, and the size and direction of these currents may be measured and recorded to help in the identification of any normal or abnormal functioning.

The tiny currents are measured by recording differences in electrical potential between pairs of electrodes attached to various parts of the body. The standard method has three pairs of electrodes wired, respectively, to the right and left arm, the right arm and left leg, and the left arm and left leg. The idea is that these provide a good general impression of the electrical activity of the heart as a whole, since they are located to pick up very characteristic signals. It is customary to supplement these three pairs with a number of other electrodes placed directly on the wall of the chest (usually in six positions); being closer to the heart, these can pick out small defects which the standard three pairs might miss, and give a more precise location to any aberration.

An ECG is often taken under controlled-exercise conditions (the exercise ECG) because this will reveal abnormalities not apparent on the resting ECG tracing. The demands on the heart and the pressure it develops are greater during exercise, so latent as well as existing CHD- or stress-related heart-rhythm disturbances may be detected.

What do the readings mean? A normal electrocardiograph will produce a printout (an

Exercise ECGs being taken.

electrocardiogram) such as you see in the diagram. Tall peaks interspersed with a regular lower one represent the muscular contractions of the heart under the control of the special pacemaker cells.

Look now at the next trace, where you can see the visual results of an over-rapid beat – tachycardia. Here the 'atrial flutter' shows as a series of fast small peaks.

In the third trace we see a similar sort of irregularity, called 'atrial fibrillation': there are sharp bursts of lower peaks, interspersed this time with fast and irregular responses from the ventricles. The atria seem to be twitching rapidly in an uncoordinated way instead of setting a steady pace for the ventricles to follow.

Should the ventricles follow suit and begin to fibrillate this is very bad news, because it usually spells the death of the individual. The ECG here looks like the fifth diagram; disorganized peaks of

ventricular activity that effectively block the action of these pumping chambers.

The electrocardiogram means as much to the cardiologist as your native tongue does to you. He can look at the peaks, troughs, rhythms and all sorts of subtleties that most of us might not notice, and see in them the 'fingerprintings' of particular kinds of disease. He may, though, want to supplement this data with information from X-rays to see whether the heart has been enlarged by disease, or he may want to go further and use more invasive methods to penetrate into the body itself. Usually this last step is not necessary, but if, for instance, it looks as if surgery may be needed, the technology is available for doctors to take a journey to the heart before an incision is made.

The cardiac catheter and contrast radiography

An essential diagnostic aid is the cardiac catheter – first developed by Werner Forssman, who conducted the dramatic experiments on himself

Today the ECG is analysed using computer technology.

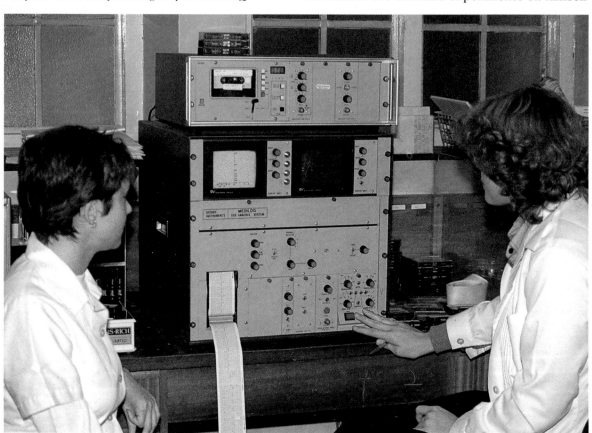

Examples of ECG Readings

A normal ECG consists of regular waves designated P, Q, R, S and T. The P wave represents current generated prior to the contraction of the atria, the QRS complex represents current generated prior to the contraction of the ventricles. The T wave is generated as the ventricles recover.

Atrial flutter. Note the irregular P waves.

Atrial fibrillation. The P waves are even more disorganized and irregular.

Complete heart block. Here there is no correlation between the occurrence of the P waves and the QRS complex.

Ventricular fibrillation. The beats are weak, irregular and disorganized – unless emergency action is taken death will rapidly ensue.

Acute anterior wall damage due to a heart attack. Note the abnormal shape of the QRS complex.

Acute posterior wall damage due to a heart attack. Again the QRS complex is grossly distorted.

Cardiac catheterization in progress.

which are described in Chapter 1. It is only because of the sophisticated development of this technique that surgery on the coronary arteries has become possible. The long, thin tube is inserted into a blood vessel in the arm and, under X-ray guidance, is gently pushed into the heart. The catheter can be fitted with a pressure-gauge, to measure the pressure in the chambers of the heart, and it is also used to collect blood samples from different areas so that their oxygen content can be measured. This information is used to diagnose the presence of septal defects and the size and direction of shunts. For example, if blood in the right atrium contains more oxygen than it should, this means that blood has shunted from the left atrium, probably through an atrial septal defect.

Another exploratory technique which uses a cardiac catheter is contrast radiography. The radiographer injects a harmless radio-opaque dye through the already positioned catheter. X-ray pictures are taken in quick succession to show the movement of the dye through the heart

and blood vessels. By positioning the catheter in different areas before injecting the dye, the cardiologist gets a clear view of the blood vessels and heart chambers – their dimensions, any obstructions, the formation of their walls and so on – enabling accurate identification of shunts and obstructions.

Radioisotopes

Another way of gathering information is to inject radioactive materials (radioisotopes), such as thallium-200, into the bloodstream. A scanner records the progress of the isotope, and thereby the blood-flow, on its journey to the heart muscle, thus providing still more information on a person's heart and circulation.

Ultrasound

Finally, there is an investigatory method which is both safe and totally noninvasive: the use of ultrasound, sound-waves of very high frequencies, far too high for us to hear. A bat beams out

A close-up showing the catheter in place. The major blood vessels can be seen quite clearly.

a

b

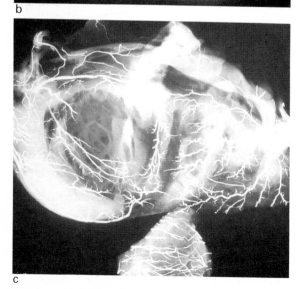

c

Coronary angiograms showing:
(a) a normal artery;
(b) coronary occlusion;
(c) myocardial infarct.

ultrasonic waves to bounce them off a likely prey, just as a warship can use ultrasound ('sonar') to detect an enemy submarine. Both bat and warship pick up the echoes, and from them can tell a great deal about the position, motion and shape of the target. In just the same way, we can bounce ultrasound off all parts of the heart, repeating this process from different positions until we have built up a picture of the shape and movement of the heart walls and valves. This technique is very similar to that used to monitor the embryo in the womb. In recent years cardiologists have been attracted to the safety and accuracy of 'ultrasound echocardiography', as it is termed in their own particular line of medical work. Taken in conjunction with the other techniques I have been discussing, it amounts to a powerful diagnostic weapon in the fight against heart disease.

THE CAUSES OF ACQUIRED HEART DISEASE

All the facts seem to be funnelling us towards one inevitable conclusion: CHD is to a large extent a man-made phenomenon. To explore that idea in detail we ought to take a trip to a small town outside Boston, Massachusetts, that lies at the heart of our current understanding of acquired coronary conditions.

The US government decided in 1948 to investigate the causes of heart disease by looking at what was deemed to be a typical small town in the USA: Framingham, a hardworking, decent community of people, mostly white and middle-class and, what was particularly useful for the investigators, very stable. Framingham folk do not, or rather did not, move about the country a lot. Thirty years after the study was started the researchers were still able to keep tabs on 80 percent of the population, which by any reckoning is quite extraordinary.

The Framingham study drew on the services of just over 5000 people – 2282 men and 2845 women (from a total population of 28 000). All

Vienna, 1950. Trial runs with radioisotopes for the diagnosis of heart disease (right).

Radioactive isotopes being packed (below).

A scan using radioactive isotopes in progress (below).

An ultrasound scan in progress (above).

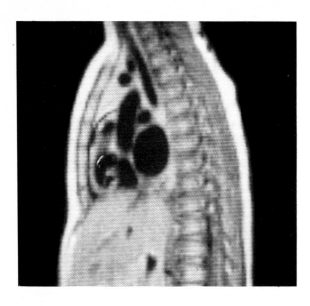

Two scans of the heart, from the side and from above.

were healthy volunteers; all were prepared to take part in an experiment that might well last as long as they did. Physical checks and tests were carried out on all of them: blood tests, ECGs to measure heart function, X-rays and blood-pressure readings and so on, and detailed medical histories on previous illnesses that they or their families had had were compiled. Once this huge initial data-gathering phase was completed, the researchers saw the 5000 every two years for re-examination, and kept in touch with the subjects' physicians on any health problems that arose. Otherwise they just sat back and waited.

Five factors associated with CHD

Over 10, 20, 30 years the participants began to die, and where possible postmortems were conducted to ascertain the causes of death in detail. The research revealed five important factors associated with death caused by CHD:

1 High blood pressure.

2 High levels of cholesterol in the blood.

3 Cigarette-smoking.

4 Glucose intolerance, such as is found in diabetics.

5 Evidence of hypertrophy (abnormal enlargement) of the left ventricle.

When these findings were first aired publicly they caused something of a sensation. Americans had at best only a vague idea of what cholesterol was, but they saw that it was doing them no good. They saw, too, that a generally fitter style of living – more exercise and fresh air, and less food, cigarettes and booze – might lessen their chances of a heart attack.

Subsequently many more studies have been carried out along similar lines to the Framingham investigation. In 1976 alone, for example, the American National Heart Institute and the American Heart Association invested a cool 400 million dollars on research into the causes of heart disease. A lot of money, until you realize that, measured in terms of hospital care, insurance claims, loss of manpower and so on, the costs of heart disease in the USA during that period totalled a staggering 58 *billion* dollars.

Since then the list of risk factors has been enlarged and refined. At the top come cigarette-smoking, hypertension (high blood pressure), and high blood cholesterol, which operate independently of any other factors. If you can admit to any of these you are at risk. Then comes a secondary list of factors that tend to operate in conjunction with others, sometimes several 'or more at a time. These include diabetes and a family history of CHD. There are also those factors that *might* increase your risk: being overweight; suffering stress; having a particular personality; being physically inactive; living in an area with hard drinking-water.

Weighing up your chances

As we have seen from the Framingham and other studies, if you are a cigarette smoker and have high levels of cholesterol in your blood and high blood-pressure, there is little doubt that you are more prone to CHD. Imagine, however – and this is very interesting to me as someone who has seen all kinds of patients over the years – that you *do* have all these factors; even so, your chances of contracting CHD in the next ten years are only one in five. Although you are in the maximum-risk category you still have an 80 percent chance of avoiding a coronary. Later on, I shall be telling you how you can make the odds even more favourable by using our new-found knowledge of the risk factors.

THE CHOLESTEROL CONTROVERSY

In January 1984 the world's media were given a full briefing on the results of an important and expensive heart study organized by the American National Heart, Lung and Blood Institute's Coronary Primary Prevention Trial, which had been begun ten years earlier. The aim of this investigation was to take many of the established findings on cholesterol and CHD one step further than the straightforward (or not so straightforward?) cause-and-effect stage.

The Framingham researchers had shown that heart disease is associated with high cholesterol levels in the blood, a strong indication that the latter was a probable cause of CHD. However, it had been by no means scientifically proven that eating a diet low in cholesterol would actually *prevent* atherosclerosis. It might seem on the face of it that it must do so, but suspicion, hunch, deduction and inference are not proof. And proof is what the National Heart, Lung and Blood Institute wanted, and was prepared to spend 150 million dollars to acquire.

The evidence

The researchers took 3806 men between the ages of 35 and 59 whom they identified as having higher than average levels of cholesterol in their bloodstream. None had signs of coronary heart disease when the study began. The subjects were split randomly into two groups: one was the test group while the other formed a control group against which the results of the test group could be evaluated.

Next, both groups were put on a low-cholesterol diet, but the test group was also

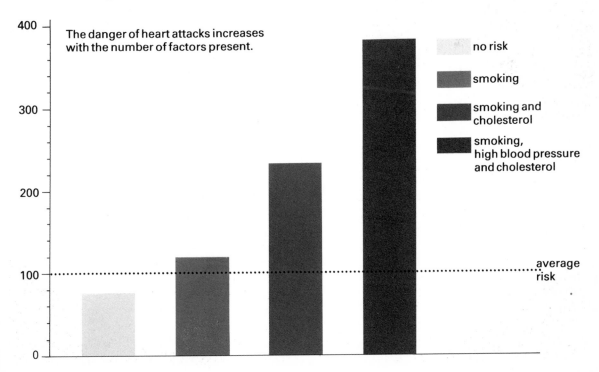

The danger of heart attacks increases with the number of factors present.

no risk

smoking

smoking and cholesterol

smoking, high blood pressure and cholesterol

average risk

given cholestyramine – a substance known to lower blood-cholesterol levels. The theory was that members of the test group should end up with less incidence of heart disease because, with the cholestyramine advantage, they were being subjected to tighter control over the amount of their cholesterol intake, particularly a type called Low Density Lipoprotein-Cholesterol (LDL-C) that reached and circulated in their bloodstream.

In the event, after nearly seven-and-a-half years on these regimes, this is exactly what

The traditional cooked breakfast is now regarded as a 'disaster diet'.

happened. Cholesterol levels dropped in both groups, but the test group had 19 percent less heart disease in general (sudden death, coronary, fatal and non-fatal heart attacks) and 24 percent fewer fatal heart attacks. There were benefits in terms of the incidence of angina and the need for coronary bypass operations.

However, we must remember that the volunteers for this trial belonged to a particularly 'at-risk' sector of the community, all having initially high LDL-C levels. In a more normal cross-section of the population it might be enough to use reduced fat diets to produce improvements. But the trial does show that, for those at risk, drugs can improve health and

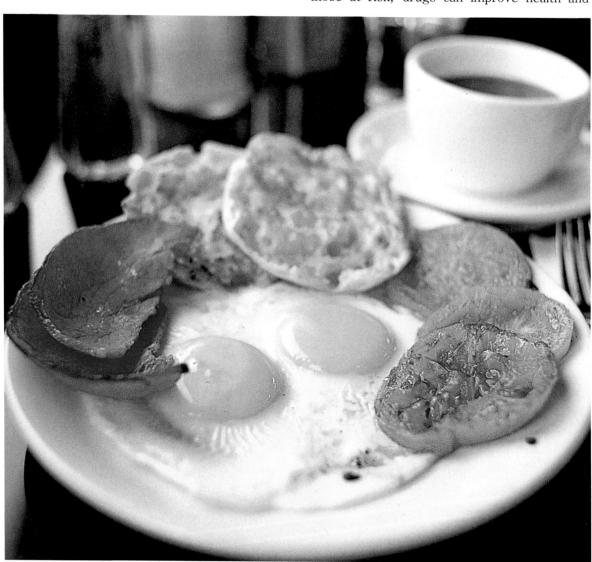

lengthen life. For every 1 percent drop in blood cholesterol the researchers found a 2 percent drop in the risk of heart attack – a very encouraging result. The research team believe that similar results could be expected among other age-groups and among women, although they have not extrapolated their results to consider people with average cholesterol levels.

The verdict

This extensive study, carried out in 12 Lipid Research Clinics, is, according to the researchers, the first to establish conclusively that lowering high blood-cholesterol in humans reduces heart attacks and deaths caused by heart attacks. For years doctors have described how excess cholesterol forms the fatty yellow substance known as 'plaque' which builds up in the cells lining the arteries. They have shown how platelets – the special protective cells that help blood coagulate – seal off these deposits, forming clots that can detach themselves from the blood-vessel wall to block blood-flow and so cause a heart attack or stroke. Now comes proof that you can improve your health by curbing directly the build-up of lipids in the first place, and probably thereby preventing deposits of fat being incorporated in the arterial wall. All very logical, you might say, even obvious – but now we have proof. *Now*, surely, we can be confident in sentencing cholesterol to exile in order to keep our hearts alive?

Well, confident perhaps, but nothing is ever simple in medicine. For example, there is some evidence that people with relatively low levels of cholesterol may be slightly more prone to cancer than those with higher levels. The issue of the relationship of lipids to malignancies is rather complicated, being tied up with the presence of Vitamin A in ways that are not fully understood.

Nevertheless, this is an interesting finding, and one which deserves further study before we start patting ourselves on the back and pretending that now we know it all. We do not.

Another complication is in determining what constitutes a high or low lipid level diet. Even a substance as fat-free as coffee can have cholesterol-related repercussions. There is evidence from studies carried out in Norway by Dr. Dag Thelle and his colleagues (*New England Journal of Medicine*, 16 June, 1983) that men drinking eight or nine cups of coffee a day have nearly 20 percent higher levels of blood cholesterol than the one-cup-a-day man. In women the lipid-level difference is 12 percent. Could imbibing coffee somehow boost blood-lipid levels? If so, does drinking coffee predispose you to coronary heart disease? The Norwegian work suggests that the answer to both questions is 'yes'. Elsewhere, and I can neither explain nor justify the inconsistencies here, researchers have come to other conclusions.

SMOKING AND HEART DISEASE

Cigarette-smoking, as everyone now recognizes, is injurious to health. Only a few beyond the fringe would argue against the proposition that smoking is linked to lung cancer. And, in the wake of the Framingham study, it is clear that cigarettes make for an unhealthy heart as well. According to the British Heart Foundation, if the entire population of the UK were to kick the smoking habit 10 000 fewer men and women of working age would die from heart attacks every year – and that figure is, by the way, higher than the number of smoking-related deaths from any other disease, including lung cancer and chronic bronchitis. Put simply, people who smoke 20 cigarettes a day are twice as likely to have a heart attack than people who smoke none. If you are over 50 the risk is a staggering 10 times greater.

So far, however, we have been talking about smoking in 'general' terms only: that such and such a cigarette consumption leads to a certain level of heart disease. What a number of researchers have been trying to find out is precisely *how* cigarette smoke causes heart problems. Probably the most important constituents in smoke in this respect are carbon monoxide (a toxic gas emitted from, among other sources, automobile exhausts) and nicotine – the active stimulant and the ingredient that gives smokers their pleasure.

Nicotine, being a stimulant, increases the production of the hormone adrenalin, which makes the heart beat faster and raises blood-pressure. Carbon monoxide, on the other hand, has a depressive effect on the vitality of the blood, because it combines with the pigment –

The following table shows that for every major cause of death, the rates for divorced males ranged anywhere from two to six times higher than those of their married counterparts.

Death rates of divorced and married men
per 100 000 population, ages 15–64 in the United States, 1959–1961

Cause of Death	White Males		Nonwhite Males	
	Married	Divorced	Married	Divorced
Heart disease	176	362	142	298
Motor vehicle accidents	35	128	43	81
Cancer of respiratory system	28	65	29	75
Cancer of digestive system	27	48	42	88
Stroke	24	58	73	132
Suicide	17	73	10	21
Cirrhosis of liver	11	79	12	53
Hypertension	8	20	49	90
Pneumonia	6	44	22	69
Homicide	4	30	51	129
Tuberculosis	3	30	15	54

haemoglobin – in the red corpuscles and impairs their capacity to transport oxygen.

The combined effects seem to be that the blood is likely to clot too freely, forming thromboses. This problem arises because smoke tends to interfere with the formation of blood platelets. A study carried out on the blood of 73 patients with coronary heart disease, as compared with a control group of 55 normal individuals, showed that the CHD group mostly had larger and denser platelets. The implication, which I find perfectly reasonable, is that the bigger the platelets the greater the likelihood of abnormal degrees of clotting, so that blockages in the coronary arteries are created.

Platelets are probably formed by the break-up of larger cells in the various blood vessels branching into the lungs after blood has been pumped there from the right ventricle for oxygenation. Smoke in the lungs impairs this fragmentation so that, instead of normal-size platelets being produced, large, sticky aggregates are generated. At the same time the

nicotine is quickening the pace of the blood-flow and the carbon monoxide is lowering the oxygen content of the blood. Cumulatively, these conditions are ideal for the creation of blockages.

For this reason I strongly recommend, if you are a smoker, heavy or light, filter or plain, cigarette or pipe, that you give it up. In Chapter 8 I shall outline one effective way of doing so.

OTHER MAJOR CAUSES OF CHD

Being too fat is associated with heart disease. If you have become overweight through excessive eating, your blood-cholesterol level will probably be raised, and of course overweight is associated with high blood-pressure. Chapter 9 will give you guidelines on correct weight and eating habits.

Before leaving this survey of causes, however, let us not forget that there is more than a grain of truth in the folk wisdom that emotional upset can be a medical liability. The term 'broken heart' can be taken both literally and figuratively, as Professor James Lynch of the

Similar changes in death rate patterns by marital status can be seen in women.

Death rates of widowed and married females
per 100 000 population, ages 15–64 in the United States, 1959–1961

Cause of Death	White females		Nonwhite females	
	Married	Widowed	Married	Widowed
Heart disease	44	67	83	165
Cancer of breast	21	21	19	28
Cancer of digestive system	20	24	25	41
Stroke	19	31	72	147
Motor vehicle accidents	11	47	10	25
Hypertensive heart disease	7	10	50	97
Cancer of cervix	7	13	17	34
Cirrhosis of liver	7	15	9	23
Suicide	6	12	3	6
Accidental fires or explosions	1	6	4	11

Source: J.J. Lynch, The Broken Heart, Basic Books, 1978

University of Maryland demonstrated so eloquently in his book with that very title – *The Broken Heart* (J. J. Lynch, Basic Books, 1978).

Dr. Lynch believes that heart disease can be linked to emotional distress caused mainly by lack of human companionship. He has been able to put together a thorough and detailed dossier of evidence to support his claim that loneliness is a coronary killer. It cannot be a coincidence, he argues spiritedly, that the incidence of premature death from heart disease is demonstrably higher among the lonely: widows, widowers, divorcees, the estranged, old people living alone, single people who socialize very little, children from broken homes. Most convincing of all, though, are the specific cases Lynch cites of the actual physical effects on the heart of a change in levels of human relationship.

Take the example of an 11-year-old girl admitted to hospital with a fractured skull and multiple injuries in the pelvis after being struck by a car. As she came out of the coma she began to show signs of considerable distress, and the ECG showed quite pronounced peaks and troughs. Then the ECG was monitored while the girl's hand was held by a comforting nurse, and during these intervals the highs and lows levelled out. When the hand was withdrawn they returned. Similarly, a man on the verge of death showed signs of ECG stabilization when the nurse was there to lend comfort, showing that it really is possible to make a direct link between the state of body and a frame of mind.

Why is it that, generally speaking, men are more prone to CHD than women? Could it be that females confer on themselves some degree of preventive protection because they are more sociable than men? Women are so often the social facilitators in the family unit, the ones who make contacts freely, while men take more time to shed their natural reserve. Women will share confidences, take an interest in others, draw to themselves a constant flow of human interaction. While this is the crudest of generalizations, it is possible that it may have something to do with the different CHD-rates between the sexes.

Chapter 4
Treating Acquired Heart Disease

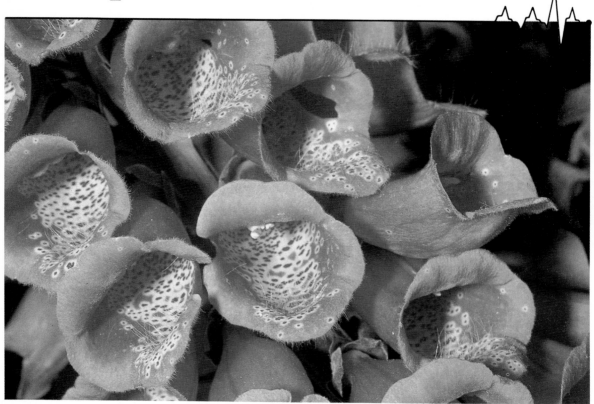

When, nearly 20 years ago, I was diagnosed as having rheumatoid arthritis, I was forced to make a rapid and profound self-appraisal. What, I wondered, do I want from life? I was to receive an answer when a rheumatologist told me that, although my condition was incurable, it would not cripple me. 'You will', he said, 'still be able to do most things'. With that prediction he gave me the most precious commodity any doctor can bestow on a patient: hope, a shred of optimism, a sense of purpose, a feeling that there is still more to come in life.

When I think of my own work as a cardiac surgeon, and all the hundreds of people who have come to me – all apprehensive, most just plain scared – that glimmer of hope is what I have always wanted to be able to give them. Fortunately, with all the modern treatments available, hope is something that heart sufferers can confidently allow themselves.

DRUGS TO COMBAT HEART FAILURE

One of the most powerful weapons in a doctor's armoury for fighting diseases of the heart, blood vessels and circulatory system is the vast range of drugs now available. There are probably over a hundred that can be prescribed, ranging from those that have been tried and tested for centuries to those that have just emerged from the biochemists' laboratories. Some are taken on their own, others used in combination. As with all powerful drugs, they should of course be used only under medical supervision.

Digitalis

1985 celebrates an important bicentenary in the history of medicine. It was 200 years ago that William Withering published a treatise on the plant that botanists know as *Digitalis purpurea*, which the rest of us recognize as the foxglove. Withering showed how the leaves of the purple foxglove could be used to make a medicinally valuable preparation that would have a tonic effect on the human heart, thus confirming something that the great herbalist Nicholas Culpeper had written more than a century earlier – a comment itself based on yet older lore.

In fact, it was not until this century that scientists managed to isolate the active constituents of digitalis extract, the cardiac glycosides which reside in the leaves of the plant. These drugs are undoubtedly among the most important heart compounds in use today. The purple foxglove, *D. purpurea*, will yield the drug digitoxin, while the white foxglove, *D. lanata,* can be used to make both digitoxin and digoxin. Incidentally, further cardiac glycosides are found in other natural homes, such as in the bulb of the sea onion.

Cardiac glycosides act by stimulating the heart to increase the force of its contractions, improving the action of the pump without increasing its oxygen consumption. At the same time, digitalis also actually slows the heart rate by acting on the vagus nerve. Overall, the drug has an effect a bit like one of those petroleum additives for cars, which raise efficiency without a corresponding increase in fuel consumption.

A failing heart produces certain key symptoms, mostly breathing disorders and an increase in fluids in various bodily tissues, called oedema ('edema' in the USA). By making the heart muscles pump more powerfully, digitalis drugs have many effects: reduced back-pressure, reduced volume of blood in the heart's chambers, and better flow of blood to the kidneys leading to improved urine output and hence a reduction in the extent of the oedema.

It is absolutely imperative that the doctor's recommended dosages of digitalis are adhered to scrupulously. For one thing it is difficult to adjust the dosages of this powerful drug to meet an individual's requirements, so once a regime has been decided upon it would be quite senseless to try to 'improve' on the prescribed amounts and frequencies. For another, digitalis, like all drugs, has certain side-effects if taken in high does. These are:

Signs of intoxication.

Headaches.

Loss of appetite.

Nausea.

Vomiting.

Diarrhoea.

Abdominal pain.

WILLIAM WITHERING, M.D. F.R.S.
FELLOW OF THE LINNÆAN SOCIETY.

William Withering (1741-1799) pioneered the use of digitalis for treating heart disease. He learned the secret of the drug from an old woman who had been using it to treat dropsy (fluid retention).

The appearance of any or some of these symptoms does not necessarily mean that you are overdosing with digitalis, but you should report any adverse effects to your doctor.

Alongside digitalis compounds, it is common for doctors to prescribe a diuretic such as chlorothiazide to maintain proper fluid levels (see later in this chapter for details of this). If so, there may be a drop in the level of potassium in your bloodstream as unusually high amounts of it are being excreted in your urine. Potassium is vital to the health of living cells, so you may also be given tablets containing this element to boost your depleted levels. Alternatively, your doctor may suggest that you take more potassium in your food; citrus fruits, bananas and most vegetables are high in potassium.

Nitrites and nitrates

The pain of angina is caused by some defect in the coronary arteries, those arteries that supply blood to the heart. Thus a substance which will

Glyceryl trinitrate or GTN is used to treat angina pain. It is available in many forms – tablets, sprays, ointments even – depending on the speed of action required. One of the fastest-acting forms is a tablet which dissolves under the tongue.

dilate blood-vessels and allow blood to flow more freely will help to relieve anginal pain.

This is precisely how nitrite and nitrate drugs work. The most important of these drugs is glyceryl trinitrate. Actually, this compound is doubly interesting because most people know it by another name and in a quite different context: it is nitroglycerine, that highly explosive basis of dynamite. Rest assured, though, that nitroglycerine as a medicine comes to you in perfectly harmless half-milligram tablets. It has a long history of success in helping angina sufferers, stretching back to the beginning of this century.

Nitrates act on the smooth muscle of the blood vessels. There, within the inner walls, they cause the muscle fibres to relax and the vessels to dilate. Blood-flow is improved, blood-pressure temporarily reduced and, within a very short space of time, pain relieved.

Unfortunately, there may be side-effects with the large doses sometimes needed to reduce the severity of angina. Headaches and flushing can occur – indeed, head pain is often difficult to avoid. High doses can also give rise to faintness if the sufferer remains on his or her feet.

Beta blockers

Another way of treating angina is by the use of one of a number of compounds – used also in the treatment of high blood-pressure – that come under the general heading of 'beta blockers'. One of the commoner examples of these is propranolol.

The heart's activity is governed by the autonomic nervous system (that part of our nervous system which controls involuntary activities such as gut movements), but in simple terms it is determined by the amount of physical work we give it to do and also by the emotional stresses we put upon it. By restricting the amount of unwanted stimulation generated by adrenalin hormones, it is possible to reduce the incidence of angina. This adrenalin stimulation is mediated by nerve-endings called beta receptors. Beta blockers shield or block the receptors and also screen the heart against excessive stimulation. If the heart is being subjected to high levels of stimulation through emotion, exercise or drugs, the beta blockers will damp down its responsiveness, slowing the rate of heart-beat

The three drugs pictured here are all beta blockers and are taken chronically, that is on a long-term management basis, to slow down heart rate. Prescription will depend on past medical history and on existing medical conditions.

Tenormin (atenolol), for example, is not contra-indicated if you happen to suffer from asthma. The pharmacological names of Inderal and Betaloc are propanolol and metoprolol respectively.

and reducing the strength of the heart's contractions, thus cutting down the amount of oxygen the heart muscle demands.

Once again – and I cannot stress this too forcefully – careful attention to your doctor's instructions as to how to take these drugs is imperative. They are not suitable for people who have suffered heart failure – indeed, they have a

slight weakening effect on heart contractions. So, unless you are also being treated for this condition, they are ruled out. The same is true if you are pregnant or have asthma or diabetes.

Side-effects of beta blockers include breathlessness and swelling of the ankles. If these are experienced, report them immediately to your doctor.

Anti-atherosclerosis drugs

Drugs for alleviating atherosclerosis – the hardening and thickening of the walls of arteries caused by deposits of fats and other substances – form another important group of compounds in the fight against heart disease. In people with high levels of blood-lipids, cholestyramine seems to reduce heart problems as it lowers blood-cholesterol, and we must assume that part of its beneficial action is due to its effect on arterial deposits. The same can be said of drugs (such as bezafibrate) which, in ways not fully understood, also lower the levels of fats and of nicotinic acid in the blood.

Anticoagulants

If the inside of a blood-vessel wall is damaged at any point a clot of blood – a thrombosis – may form at this site; the clot may stay where it is, impeding the blood-flow, or move on around the body to cause what is called an embolism. Coronary thrombosis is the result of an unwanted aggregation of clotted blood. Drugs designed to interfere with, and sometimes prevent, clotting are called 'anticoagulants'.

These drugs fall into two main groups. First come substances such as heparin which directly assist in preventing blood from clotting; these are administered by injection into the blood-stream. Second are the oral anticoagulants, such as nicoumalone and warfarin, which are taken in tablet form and act indirectly by stopping the body from producing one of its numerous 'clotting factors'.

Anticoagulants like heparin slow down the process of clotting. Heparin can be highly effective, but again it is not without side-effects: bleeding from the nose, bruising, and sometimes fever and allergy. Doctors like to monitor the progress of the clotting times in a patient very closely, both to adjust the dosage if required and, on occasions, to try to discontinue treatment altogether.

The indirect anticoagulants are mainly derivatives of a substance called coumarin. Their action is a good deal slower than that of the direct-action drugs, perhaps taking several days to be effective; for this reason, if there is any sense of urgency in the case, heparin is frequently prescribed initially. Again careful checks on how

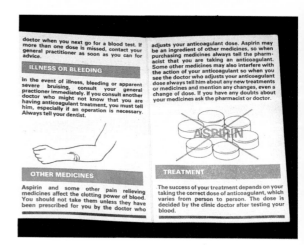

A warning about taking aspirin – either per se *or as an ingredient of other medicines – while taking anticoagulants.*

long clotting is taking are necessary, and adverse effects, mainly bleeding, are not unknown.

In short, anticoagulants should be taken with extreme caution, and strictly in accordance with your physician's advice. There are a number of reasons why you might not be able to take the drugs – impaired kidney function, having just had a baby, recovering from surgery, taking other drugs and so on. In fact, patients on anticoagulant therapy are usually given a warning card to carry so that doctors can take this into account when prescribing further drug treatments.

If a blood clot has formed there are drugs available to help dissolve it. One of these is streptokinase, which is an enzyme, or biological catalyst. The drug is administered either by an intravenous injection or by means of a catheter snaked directly into the coronary artery where the clot has formed. This is, of course, a delicate business, and to be effective the procedure has to be carried out very soon after a warning sign has indicated that coronary thrombosis is the problem. Conversely, the risks are comparatively small and the advantages for people with a high risk of acute heart attack are undeniable. Streptokinase, although still experimental, has reduced the likelihood of death resulting from a first or second heart attack.

Anticoagulants are essential drugs for people who have been fitted with mechanical heart-valve replacements.

Diuretics

Most diuretics act on the kidneys to increase the body's output of sodium salts and water in the urine. This can have considerable therapeutic benefits. If the heart is not working efficiently the capacity of the kidneys to excrete salts is impaired, and this in turn means that the body retains more fluid in order to dissolve the resultant salt-overload. Diuretics such as those in the thiazide group act to raise both salt- and

A selection of diuretic preparations to help the body get rid of water and salt. They are especially valuable in heart patients with congestion of the lungs; poor oxygen absorption by waterlogged lungs puts strain on the heart. Some of these agents are potassium-sparing – they prevent the loss of too much potassium in the urine; others contain a potassium supplement to replace potassium lost in the urine. Navidrex-K below is one such (K is the chemical symbol for potassium).

water-output by preventing the kidneys from reabsorbing salt from the urine back into the bloodstream. One snag is that, in the process, the kidneys also make the body shed too much potassium, so this deficit has to be made good, especially since one effect of a potassium deficit is to weaken the heart. Sometimes both functions can be performed by a drug that combines the action of a diuretic with that of a potassium conserver.

There is a wide range of diuretics from which your doctor can choose, varying in speed of action, potency and side-effects. So far as adverse reactions are concerned, you should watch out for any of the following and report them to your doctor: nausea, dizziness, rashes, numbness, pins and needles, and allergic reactions. Patients on diuretics should sensibly control their fluid and salt intakes.

Drugs to set the proper rhythm

There are many ways in which the heart's natural and proper rhythm can be disrupted, and there is a correspondingly large armoury of drugs available to combat these arrhythmias. Among the drugs used to treat rhythm disorders are quinidine, desopyramide, rhythmodan, verapamil and bretylium. Also used are procainamide (a relative of the local anaesthetic, procaine), lignocaine (another local anaesthetic, used to set right a short-term disorder), phenytoin (used for many years to treat epileptic fits but more recently for heart-rhythm disorders), and beta-blockers which, as we have seen, act on the autonomic nervous system to induce calm. As these drugs all have different modes of action, the choice of the particular drug which you will be prescribed will depend on the type of rhythm disorder from which you are suffering.

Side-effects are again possible and problematical: they include rashes, headaches, sore throats, vomiting, cramp and diarrhoea. Again, see your doctor should any of these occur.

Unusual remedies

Alongside conventional drug treatments is a whole range of 'alternative' methods; some of these are endorsed quite enthusiastically by doctors, others are not. My own view is a combination of open-mindedness and question-

Lanoxin is one of many preparations containing digoxin, derived from digitalis from the humble floxglove. Digoxin helps to control arrhythmias.

ing scepticism. If an alternative remedy is put forward as 'working' or 'being useful' in acquired heart disease, I want to see the evidence and judge it with the same hard-headedness as I would any other therapy. But I do not rule anything out just because at first sight it seems to be unorthodox. After all, in the early days, heart transplants were an ambitious sort of technique until people realized their undoubted value.

Here are some of the less conventional approaches to drug therapy:

Vitamin E. According to Dr. Wilfrid E. Shute in his book *Vitamin E for Ailing and Healthy Hearts* (Pyramid House, 1969) Vitamin E helps to prevent coronary thrombosis. It does this by stopping blood clots from forming, and will even help dissolve them if they have already formed. Dr. Shute argues that the rise of cardiovascular disease in the USA coincided with the widespread adoption of the practice of milling wheat into refined white flour, a process which effectively removes the major source of Vitamin E in flour, the wheat germ. So far there has not been a large-scale controlled study on Vitamin E and heart disease, comparable to that on dietary fats, so we must not jump to conclusions too readily. But it is an interesting idea.

Vitamin C. There has been a lot of publicity surrounding this vitamin in recent years, mainly because of its suggested role in staving off infection. However Dr. R. Hume and his colleagues at the Southern General Hospital in Glasgow showed that in the acute phase of a heart attack levels of Vitamin C (ascorbic acid) in the bloodstream fall dramatically (R. Hume *et al.*, *British Heart Journal*, Vol. 34, 1972.). Where then does the Vitamin C go? If it makes its way to the heart to help to repair the tissue damaged by oxygen deprivation, perhaps Vitamin C may also be used as a preventive measure, stopping emergencies from erupting. Further research is needed to explore this possibility.

Hard and soft water. People sing the praises of soft water but there is evidence that it may not be preferable to the hard variety so far as cardiovascular disease is concerned. According to an article in the *Lancet* by Drs. Crawford, Gardner and Morris (1971, ii, pp. 327-29), in those towns where the water is hard (that is, with relatively high levels of calcium and magnesium in the water) death rates from cardiovascular disease are lower than in soft-water areas. In other words, it could be that calcium and magnesium help to prevent acquired heart disease. On the other hand, it could be that soft water contains certain elements that may be injurious to health.

'Natural foods'. Here there are many candidates for an 'anti-heart disease' remedy and I do not propose to go into all of them. Suffice it to say that, for every one genuinely interesting suggestion, there are probably about ten times as many outright cranky ones. Among the more recent ideas is the notion that pectin, a carbohydrate found in the cell walls of many vegetables and fruits, may limit the amount of cholesterol the body can absorb. Which is why

Drs. Hans Fisher and Paul Priminger suggest in *Farm Journal* (April 1968) that an apple a day really does keep the doctor away. I am not aware of any detailed research into the benefits of pectin, but here is surely a case of a remedy that, if taken in moderation, will no no harm.

But a word of warning. Never take any alleged 'natural cure' to excess by eating vast quantities of foods said to be 'good for you'. There comes a point when even a benign product such as an apple or a carrot can actually become dangerous if ingested in too great a quantity and at the expense of all other foods. An imbalanced diet is, medically, a bad thing, not to mention the monotony of single-food programmes.

There are numerous other suggestions for 'alternative' cures, such as aspirin, tea and fish oil, but until these are fully investigated in properly run, scientifically sound studies, they should be treated with caution. Certainly, anyone with a heart condition should try them only after discussion with a physician.

Which drug for which condition?

There is no such thing as *the* drug for *the* condition, because we all react differently to different substances. So, while the news may perhaps dismay some of you, I am forced to stress that the age-old process of trial and error comes into the clinical picture here. A doctor has to be sensitive to what is going on within his patient. He may start with one drug, and then abandon it altogether in favour of another. Or he may supplement the original drug with a different compound that helps offset, for example, a particular side-effect. Or he may decide that drugs, except for use in certain emergencies, are less beneficial than lifestyle changes, such as in diet or exercise.

Whatever route is taken, go along with it. What you can do to help, though, is keep a very watchful eye open for side-effects, which should be explained by your doctor when prescribing a heart drug for you. What they are, how severe and how long-lasting – all such information might be relevant, and should be duly noted. Take all the details along to your physician as soon as possible and do something that will stand you both in good stead: talk.

SURGERY FOR ACQUIRED HEART DISEASE

In practice, heart surgery – while it will never be a commonplace routine like removing ingrown toe-nails – has become a tried, tested and safe means of alleviating sickness and saving lives. It is true that surgery may not be attempted until a regime of drugs or lifestyle changes has been tried, but, on the other hand, with modern diagnostic procedures doctors can often spot straight away those individuals who would benefit from immediate surgery.

It must always be remembered that surgery for acquired heart disease is mainly palliative rather than curative, and therefore should be resorted to only when patients have symptoms and signs that show that their condition can be alleviated by the procedure. The most common operations are for acquired diseases of the valves and coronary arteries – the latter is sometimes called ischemic heart disease or myocardial ischemia.

CORONARY ARTERY SURGERY

If diagnostic tests indicate a blockage in the coronary arteries the commonest remedial measure is the coronary-artery bypass – although as early as the 1950s, my colleagues and I were exploring other methods of improving blood-supply to the heart. Experiments on dogs using the mammary artery were successful: we joined the mammary artery to the coronary artery and then ligated (tied-off) the coronary artery. These were some of the first experiments in direct revascularizing of the heart muscle.

It is estimated that in the USA 120 000 people a year undergo coronary-bypass surgery, a procedure pioneered in the early 1960s by Dr. Michael DeBakey and Dr. Edward Garrett of Houston. They first removed a section of a patient's leg-vein and used it as a graft to bypass a clogged section of artery, promptly relieving the pain of angina and allowing the patient to survive another nine years.

Subsequently Dr. DeBakey carried out a study following up the outcome of bypass surgery on 3500 patients. He found that over 80

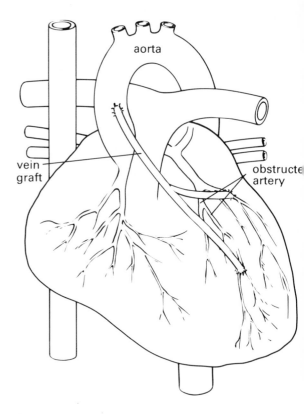

Coronary-artery bypass. The number of grafts inserted depends on how many coronary arteries are obstructed. The graft passes directly from the aorta to beyond the obstruction in each artery so that the blood supply to the heart is increased.

percent survived ten years or so after surgery, with half of those under the age of 65 working full-time. In other countries bypass surgery, although regularly performed, is less popular than in the USA. In the UK, for example, it seems that only one operation is carried out for every 12 in the USA, per capita; the Swiss come somewhere in the middle. Why these national differences should exist is a difficult question. The operations are not especially cheap to undertake, and not all doctors agree about the life-prolonging effects of a bypass. Still others argue that resources are better channelled into preventive measures, the bypass being only a palliative procedure, doing nothing to strike at the root cause of the disease. And so the debate continues.

It has to be said that, because this operation is a money-spinner, it can be over-used, like tonsillectomies were 20 years ago. The most important indication that a bypass operation is desirable is uncontrollable angina; where there are only minor symptoms, the operation should be carried out only if there is evidence of other life-threatening lesions, such as an obstruction of the main left coronary artery. But I have to qualify this by saying that, if I had uncontrollable angina due to blocked arteries, I would move heaven and earth to get into the operating theatre – particularly as the hospital mortality rate for this operation is very low (less than one percent).

The bypass operation

For the operation the patient is of course anaesthetized, with the heart-lung machine standing by ready to take over during the critical phase of the grafting. A non-essential vein is removed from the patient's own leg (no rejection problems here) and one end of it is stitched into

A bypass operation. The graft is being made ready for implantation.

position in front of the blockage (i.e., on the side farthest away from the heart). The other end of the vein is then sewn directly into the aorta, thus producing a bypass around the blockage and allowing blood to flow freely from the aorta into the heart. Not just one, but several bypasses can be fashioned in a single operation. In order to perform the delicate stitching, the surgeon needs a quiet heart (i.e., one that is not beating), and so a cold, heart-paralysing solution is injected into the coronary system after the patient has been put on the heart-lung machine. To start the heart again after the work has been completed, warm blood is allowed to flow back into the coronary system. Usually the heart begins to beat spontaneously, but sometimes it needs artificial electrical stimulation to nudge it back to life.

As for results, more than nine out of ten people get some relief from symptoms with a bypass operation and six out of ten get total relief. There is no doubt that the quality of life of the patient is enhanced by the operation, which allows a chance to return to a level of physical

The first coronary-artery bypass was done in 1969 at London's Brompton Hospital. Mr. Edward Timson is pictured here after the operation – a month previously he could not walk without fighting for breath.

activity that previously had been out of the question. I well remember the second patient on whom I performed this operation. His angina was so severe that he was taking *eighty* nitroglycerine tablets a day. After the operation he had no angina at all.

After the operation a few rules and regulations are to be expected. Your doctor will probably put you on a course of drugs. Physical exercise must be taken carefully to start with, so that you build up your levels of exertion very gradually, and, if you feel like it, punctuate your day with a rest in bed. You may get a few aches and pains in your chest and leg – after all, your chest has been opened up for the operation and this will take time to heal, as will the vein wound in your leg.

At night you may sweat a little. Driving is out for the immediate post-op period but can be resumed after about six weeks. Sex is all right, but be sensible and avoid ultra-strenuous activity until your general level of exertion is around normal again. As for work, research shows that more than half of all bypass patients are back on blockage is first identified, and then the artery is opened and the plaque dissected away from the wall, using a blunt instrument or a fine jet of carbon dioxide gas. I describe other more experimental procedures in Chapter 6.

SURGERY FOR VALVE DISEASE

As I mentioned in Chapter 1, there are various causes of valve malfunction, such as rheumatic fever, atherosclerosis *in* the valves, syphilis or other viral and bacterial infections or congenital defects. The two heart valves most likely to succumb to disease are the important inlet and outlet valves on either side of the left ventricle, the mitral and aortic valves. If the damage is severe and surgery is required then there are two strategies available: repair or replacement. In practice, repair is virtually never possible for the aortic valve and so a replacement is the only choice. There are more available options in the case of the mitral valve, depending on the nature of the disease and how far it has progressed. With the improvement in the types of artificial valves available, repair procedures are becoming more and more unpopular (except in mitral stenosis without calcification).

Once it is decided that a replacement valve is needed, there are two choices: either one can opt for a mechanical valve, such as the Starr, Björk-Shilley or Saint Jude; or one can choose to use a valve made of biological materials. Whichever type of valve is inserted, the risk of mortality is low, around three to five percent, which is about the same as that for major abdominal surgery.

Mechanical valves

Mechanical valves have several advantages. They are readily available in a variety of sizes, easily sterilized, haemodynamically adequate and durable. However, people with mechanical valves have to take anticoagulants for the rest of their lives to prevent clots forming around the artificial materials, and this means a trip to hospital every six to eight weeks – a grave problem if you live in a remote area. Another drawback is that some types of mechanical valves make a clicking noise. I remember a sad story about a patient of mine who had been fitted

the treadmill within 12 weeks of their operation, and more than eight out of ten by the end of one year. Take advice from your doctor if you are in one of those trades – like driving heavy vehicles – where stresses are known to be severe.

Alternatives to a bypass

Not all blockages in the coronary arteries are dealt with by a bypass grafting operation. Doctors have been attempting a number of other procedures for coping directly with the arterial obstructions, such as endarterectomy, the removal of the plaque-sealed obstruction from the inner wall of the artery. The site of the

A mechanical valve is inserted to replace the mitral valve.

The real thing. Open-heart surgery showing the implantation of a replacement valve.

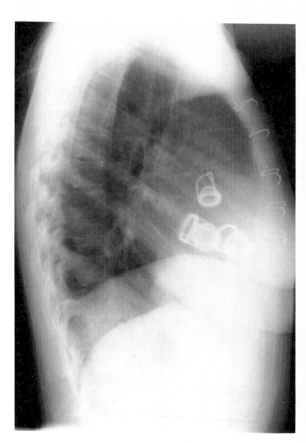

An X-ray showing a heart with three artificial valves. Note also the wire sutures holding the breast-bone together.

Making an artificial heart valve from synthetic material.

with one of these valves. One evening he was sitting quietly with his wife, when he realized that he could no longer hear the noise. He stood up and said to his wife, 'My heart has stopped', and then he died.

The history of the development of these mechanical valves is fascinating, but beyond the scope of this book. I wrote my thesis for my Master of Science degree on research I did into the development of artificial valves and the flow of blood through them. The University of Cape Town (UCT) valve which I worked on was a refinement of the Starr-Edward valve, in that it was far less bulky.

Biological valves

Biological valves, which have been used widely only in the last twenty years, come from a variety of sources: the aortic valves of pigs, the pericardium of calves, and valves from human donors. Using the patient's own tissue has been abandoned because, surprisingly, there was a much higher incidence of fibrosis and calcification. The biological material is treated to make it more durable and more readily accepted by the host's immune system.

Biological valves have the advantage of being silent, and patients fitted with them do not need anticoagulants. However, they are definitely less durable than their mechanical counterparts, so are not fitted in patients under the age of 40.

OTHER KINDS OF REPAIR WORK

The bypass and valve repair or replacement are the major surgical contributions to fighting acquired heart disease, but they are by no means the only ones. Undoubtedly the most spectacular contribution is in the treatment of aneurysm. Sometimes after a heart attack the scar tissue created during the attack may become weakened by the constant beating of the muscle, so that the wall begins to swell up like the inner tube bulging out of a bicycle tyre. After a time this swelling or aneurysm may reach quite large proportions. The first time such an aberration was operated on, in 1931, it was by mistake. The celebrated surgeon Ferdinand Sauerbruch thought that his patient had a large cystic tumour in her chest cavity. When he inserted a needle, out spurted blood rather than the expected contents of a tumour, so he hastily tried to stem the flow by sewing up the needle-hole. This just made things worse. 'Suddenly', he narrated, 'a strong column of blood spurted from the mistaken cyst sac. I rapidly introduced my index and middle fingers into the open wound and stopped the flow of blood. Quickly I had an assistant pass two strong

Some different types of replacement valves.

silk ligatures – the bleeding ceased.' It was not a tumour, then, but an aneurysm of the ventricle.

This dangerous bulge, which can occur also in the aorta, can easily be removed by surgery. The patient is connected to a heart-lung machine and his or her heart is stopped by cooling and the administration of a cardioplegic solution. The fibrous tissue of the aneurysm is cut away and the opening closed up by suturing. Once the patient's own heart is pumping again the blood flows normally through the ventricle.

Another rarer condition which can be surgically treated is a tumour in the heart, which can now be removed.

NEW HEARTS FOR OLD

In some conditions, however, the heart itself is so intrinsically diseased that repair just is not possible. Even with all the skill available to him, the surgeon cannot produce a viable organ by adding bits or taking pieces away if the original is damaged beyond repair. An analogy is trying to repair a threadbare jacket by cutting bits off and adding patches: there comes a time when it simply will not work. What is required in the case of a 'threadbare' heart is a new one – a heart transplant.

The right patient

Not everyone whose heart is irreparably damaged can have a transplant. Apart from obvious considerations like a shortage of donors, operating times and resources are limited and, therefore, decisions have to be made to select some patients and reject others. 'Doctors playing God' is the phrase which the media throw at surgeons for performing this unhappy task but, unfortunately, nobody else seems willing (or able) to do it and hence this onerous and upsetting role falls on us.

The ideal patient for a heart transplant is under 40, has severe cardiac failure untreatable by any other method, and has no evidence of disease in any other organ. However, such a perfect candidate is the exception rather than the rule, so most of the selection criteria we use are relative. But there are also some absolutes: patients with active infection, diabetes mellitus or malignancy cannot be considered for the operation because the drugs used for post operative immunosuppression will cause these conditions to deteriorate dramatically. Other disorders, such as an active peptic ulcer, chronic bronchitis and emphysema, peripheral or cerebral vascular disease and dysfunction of other major organs such as the liver and the kidneys are undesirable but are not in themselves necessarily contraindications to heart transplantation.

A point to remember is that treatment does not stop when the patient is discharged from hospital, but must be continued for the rest of his or her life. It is vitally important, therefore, that the intended recipient is psychologically and emotionally stable, and willing and able to comply with the complex drug regime and regular hospital attendances which will become an important and routine feature of his or her life once the initial excitement has died down.

The right donor

In much the same way that not everyone is suited to be a transplant recipient, so not every heart offered is suitable for implantation. Criteria that are often remarkably similar to those for the intended recipient are applied.

Obviously pre-existing cardiac disease excludes the use of a heart. In this instance one would be merely swapping one set of problems for another. The major source of donor hearts is from people dying of a head injury or a spontaneous intra-cranial haemorrhage. Age is an important consideration, with 45 being the approximate upper cut-off point; above this age, atheroma in the coronary arteries is more likely, although if there is any doubt coronary arteriography can be performed. Transferable diseases, such as infections and malignancy, along with diabetes mellitus and hypertension would render a potential donor heart unsuitable.

A blood sample is taken from the donor to check for bacterial infections, syphilis and hepatitis B. While the transplant operation is not delayed pending these results they are, if positive, of considerable importance in the follow-up care of the recipient. In addition the donor's tissue is 'typed' so that all relevant information is available in the event of a transplant.

Care of the donor and removal of the heart

Lay people usually believe that preparing the donor heart for transplantation is an easy step, that it is simply removed from the thorax and stored in ice until it is needed. Nothing could be further from the truth. The medical and surgical skills required to keep the donor heart in optimum condition are at least as great as those required for the successful transplantation itself.

Inevitably, because of the patient's condition, mechanical ventilation will have been employed, and this will be continued after brain-death has been diagnosed. Even now, large volumes of urine will be passed and there will be a danger of depletion of the circulatory volume unless fluid, and occasionally blood, is replaced intravenously. Through these drip lines the central venous pressure is monitored and drugs such as antibiotics, vasoconstrictors or heart stimulants can be given if required. In fact, the whole management technique is very similar to that given to any patient in the intensive-care unit. In this way the heart can be maintained in a viable condition for several hours, occasionally up to 24 hours, before the inevitable onset of increasing circulatory instability.

At this stage mention should be made of the donor's relatives, who are going through an extremely harrowing and anxious time. Although many are comforted by the knowledge that their loss may enable someone else to benefit, we all – not just the particular recipient – owe them a debt of gratitude which can never be repaid.

The donor is taken to the operating theatre under the care of an anaesthetist who ensures that his circulatory, respiratory and renal functions are adequately maintained. An incision is made and the heart inspected visually for signs of major damage due to trauma or external cardiac massage. The major blood vessels are cut, freeing the heart and enabling it to be removed in its entirety, a procedure taking five to ten minutes from beginning to end. The heart can then be immediately transplanted or, if it is necessary to transport it, stored in ice for up to 12 hours, a period which can be extended to up to 48 hours if more complex preservation methods are used.

Overleaf: The Papworth transplant method.

The heart transplant operation

Since donor and recipient are rarely at the same location, the timing of donor heart removal and recipient preparation must be very carefully co-ordinated. As soon as brain-stem death of the donor has occurred, the heart is maintained in a viable condition by being placed in circuit with a life support machine. As soon as the heart has been surgically exposed, it is rapidly cooled, arrested in diastole so that it holds a sufficient quantity of oxygenated blood, and excised at the roots of the major inflow and outflow vessels just above their respective valves.

When being made ready for transit, it is immersed in a cardioplegic solution at about 2°C, and placed in a cool-box.

By the time the donor heart arrives at the operating theatre, the recipient's thoracic cavity has been opened by mid-sternum split and the rib-cage is held open by retractors secured to a frame on the operating table.

The recipient has been cannulated ready for by-pass and is on a life support machine. The pericardium has been incised longitudinally on the midline and sutured to the edges of the cavity wound to provide a well for cold saline, used to protect the transplant by local cooling.

The great vessels and the atrial walls of the recipient's heart are now dissected. Incisions are made in the left and right atria of the donor heart, in such a way that they can be sutured to the residue of the atrial walls of the recipient.

PREPARATION OF RECIPIENT

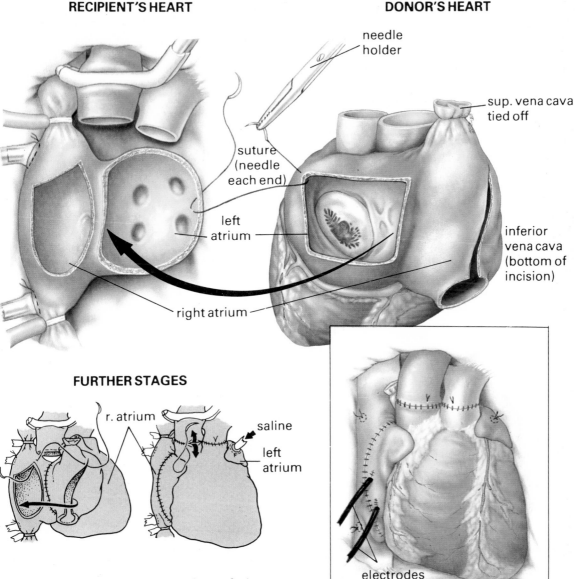

RECIPIENT'S HEART

DONOR'S HEART

needle holder

sup. vena cava tied off

suture (needle each end)

left atrium

inferior vena cava (bottom of incision)

right atrium

FURTHER STAGES

r. atrium

saline

left atrium

electrodes

COMPLETED OPERATION

Further stages in the suturing of the donor heart to the residue of the recipient's are shown above. During the final stage, aortic anastomosis, the left heart is flushed out with saline through a catheter in the left atrium to remove as much air as possible before actual closure of the aorta. Expulsion of any vestige of air remaining is achieved by placing the patient in a particular position and creating a needle hole in the ascending aorta.

Before the pericardium is sutured into place over the new heart, two electrodes are secured into positions in the right atrium wall as a temporary measure, to assist 'pacing' of the heart once the patient has been removed from the life support machine, and to provide the best connection for an ECG. The shape of the R-wave of the electrocardiograph is the earliest reliable indication of any graft rejection, should this occur.

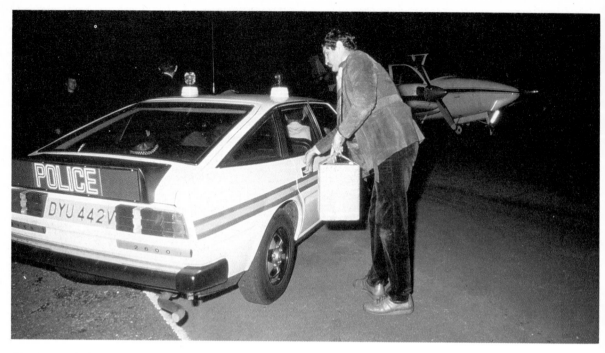

The drama of a heart transplant. A police car waits at
Elstree aerodrome in the UK for a donor heart to be flown in
from Holland.

As soon as it was known that a compatible heart was
available the recipient, John Wade, was prepared for the
operation, to be carried out by Magdi Yacoub, world-famous
heart surgeon, at Harefield Hospital (below).

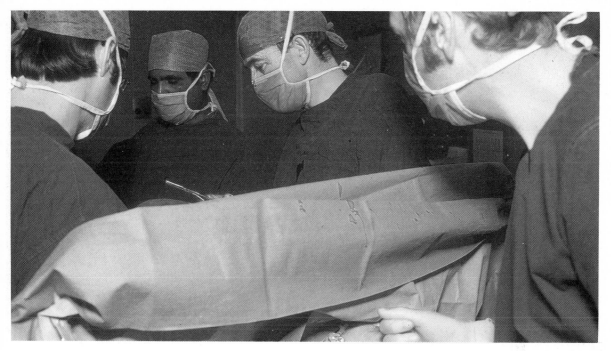

The heart-lung machine is connected so that John's brain and body have a continuous supply of fresh oxygenated blood, even though his heart is no longer pumping.

Exactly 2 hours and 56 minutes after the donor heart has been removed, it arrives in the operating theatre at Harefield (below).

Mr. Yacoub holds the donor heart above John's open chest and sizes it up. John's own heart is still in place. The donor heart will be trimmed ready for implantation – once all is ready the old heart will be removed.

It has taken over two hours to get the new heart in place. Each joint is checked for leaks, after the heart has been shocked into rhythm. The chest cavity can now be closed.

Three days later . . . John on an exercise bike. Four days later he walked nearly five miles. Before the operation he could barely walk twenty-five yards.

The transplant

The cells and tissues of every person have a genetic make-up which is specific to that individual – a 'genetic fingerprint', if you like. When a donor heart becomes available it must be matched as closely as possible to the genetic constitution of the recipient. This process is known as tissue-typing. In a way, the name is misleading since the tests are done wholly on blood: no actual heart-tissue is removed for testing. In addition to very accurate ABO blood group matching, we also try to match substances called human leucocyte antigens (HLA); these give rise to the immune response which leads to transplant rejection. Also important are tests for preformed or *cytotoxic* antibodies, which might not be compatible with the recipient's tissue. Every potential heart-transplant recipient has already been tissue-typed and the details logged on a central computer. When a donor heart becomes available the donor's HLA status is assessed and compared with those stored on the computer to get as close a match as possible.

A potential recipient is then identified and prepared for the operation. The use of antibiotics and immunosuppressant drugs is started at this stage. Following a general anaesthetic the chest is opened and the heart exposed. The patient is now put on a cardiopulmonary bypass machine (heart-lung machine), which takes over the functions of the heart and lungs until the new heart is pumping satisfactorily.

To remove the recipient's own heart incisions are made in such a way that cuffs of the atrial walls are left to allow easy suturing of the donor heart; the aorta and pulmonary artery are divided as close to their respective valves as possible. The donor heart can then be placed in the recipient's chest and joined to the patient's own circulatory system. By the time the final stitches are being put in the pulmonary artery, the new heart has usually already started contracting either rhythmically or in ventricular fibrillation. If fibrillation occurs, the usual defibrillation techniques are used.

An alternative to replacing the entire heart (orthotopic heart transplant) is to place the donor heart alongside the recipient's own and joined to it in such a way that blood can pass through either or both hearts. This is a heterotopic or 'piggy-back' transplant. Both hearts will then pump blood at their own rate without adversely affecting each other's performance.

This technique has the advantage that, if rejection of the new heart occurs, the patient's circulation can be maintained at least for a certain length of time by the patient's own heart while other steps are taken to improve the situation.

While the entire operation can last between five and nine hours, the actual transplantation itself takes only about one hour. The patient is nearly always conscious when he or she returns to the intensive-care unit. Because of the immunosuppression therapy, meticulous care must be taken to avoid introducing infection, but otherwise the post-operative care of a heart-transplant patient is the same as that for any other patient who has undergone open-heart surgery. Passive muscle exercises of the legs are begun within two hours of the operation; within 48 hours the patient will be standing out of bed and within three or four days static dynamic bicycle-riding will be started for up to one hour daily. When one considers that because of their cardiac failure most of these patients will have been relatively inactive or even bedridden for weeks or months before the operation, the magnitude of this achievement becomes readily apparent.

Problems of rejection

With the tying of the last suture, the first phase of the heart-transplant is completed. The task of preventing the recipient's body from rejecting its new heart must now begin.

Although detailed tests were carried out to find the recipient whose tissue-type most closely resembled that of the heart to be transplanted, a perfect match (except in the case of identical twins) is never possible. The recipient's body identifies the new heart as 'not self', and his or her immune system is activated to isolate and destroy the invader just as it does with any infecting virus or bacterium which manages to penetrate the body's outer defence mechanisms. Left to itself, the immune system would succeed in its objective with ruthless efficiency and speed. To prevent this happening, drugs are given to damp-down or suppress the normal immune response.

Previously, immunosuppressant drugs such as azathiaprine, cyclophosphamide and anti-thymocyte globulin were used, but these have now largely been superseded by Cyclosporin-A, in combination with low-dose corticosteroids. Relatively large doses are given in the months immediately after the operation, but these are gradually reduced to a suitable maintenance dosage, tailored individually for each patient. The drug treatment will never be stopped. Rejection has occurred as long as five years after transplantation in a patient who stopped taking his medications.

Through the suppression of the immune system, the body's defences as a whole are effectively neutralized, and the patient becomes susceptible to any passing infection. Because of this the patient is tended in a clean-air environment with nurses, doctors and relatives changing into operating-theatre gowns before entering the room. Subsequently precautions can be reduced as the recipient's body adapts to the presence of the new organ but, at all stages, a compromise must be reached between the need to prevent rejection and the possibility of overwhelming infection because of the patient's reduced ability to resist it.

Is it worth it?

Having read about the operation and the difficulties of preventing rejection, one is entitled to ask: 'Is it worth it?' I believe that the answer must be an overwhelming 'yes'. Remember, these are patients whose death is nigh because of a failing heart and for whom no other treatment will work. Without a heart transplant they would die within weeks or, at longest, months. For me though, the value of transplants is not so much that they prolong life, but that they improve the quality of a patient's life immeasurably.

Improvements in patient selection, management and immunosuppression, particularly the advent of Cyclosporin-A, have produced significant improvements in survival rates. At the present time, two of my patients have survived for more than 12 years after their operation while another three remain alive after eight years. Sadly, most are not so fortunate, but even so recent reports show one- and two-year survival rates of 65 to 80 percent while between 28 and 44 percent of patients will still be alive four years after transplantation, figures which compare favourably with those for routinely performed operations in our hospitals today.

Deaths, when they occur, are usually due to either infection or rejection of the heart. Results from different centres show the dual problem of immunosuppression very clearly: in general, those centres with an aggressive policy of immunosuppression have a higher incidence of patients dying from infection, while rejection of the transplant is the commonest cause of death in those hospitals which adopt a more conservative approach.

As the drugs used to combat rejection improve and greater public awareness leads to more donor hearts becoming available, heart transplantation will become an increasingly common and cost-effective method of treating people for whom the only alternative is a certain and imminent death.

Heart–lung transplants

Some people with congenital heart problems, such as the Eisenmenger type of 'blue baby', cannot be helped by a new heart alone. Over time, their condition will have had deleterious effects on the blood vessels in their lungs, and so what is called for is a heart–lung transplant. The development of this procedure has only been made possible by the anti-rejection drug Cyclosporin-A, which does not make a patient quite as susceptible to infection as do other similar drugs. This has meant that heart–lung operations can now be tackled with some serious hope of success, albeit only with the sort of limited results that I had for the first few heart-alone transplants.

THE POSTOPERATIVE CARE OF CARDIAC SURGERY CASES

Surgery on the heart, either replacing damaged arteries or valves or involving much more complex reconstruction work, was until relatively recently a new and exciting innovation carried out at a few major specialist centres. Now it is so commonplace that these procedures form a routine part of the operating day in most large district general hospitals. While the success of

How rejection is spotted

The most difficult part of heart transplantation is the meticulous aftercare which is necessary to prevent the rejection of the new heart by the recipient's immune mechanisms and to control infection. For the first few weeks after the transplant the patient lives on a knife-edge: too light a drug regime and he will reject the donor heart, too heavy a regime and he will become highly vulnerable to infection.

The invention of a technique for taking tissue specimens from the living heart has been crucial to the success of heart transplantation. The biopsy is performed using a tiny grab (bottom picture) on the end of a long wire which is inserted into the jugular vein in the neck and pushed down gently right into the heart, closely monitored by X-ray. Once in the heart, the grab is opened and, when it touches the heart wall (this is signalled by the completion of an electric circuit), its jaws are closed, nipping off a tiny specimen of heart muscle.

The specimen is stained and microscopically examined by Dr. Ariela Pomerance at Mount Vernon Hospital, Middlesex in England. When the heart is actively rejected there is an increase in invading cells (lymphocytes) whose job is to destroy foreign matter in the body. The middle picture shows such an increase in lymphocytes (dyed dark blue): more drugs must be given urgently. (The top picture shows normal heart muscle.)

Mr. Yacoub says: 'The first two or three months are the most dangerous time for rejection. In time the immune system adapts to the foreign heart. We don't understand how'.

Source: The Sunday Times Colour Supplement, 19 October 1981.

the heart operation is primarily determined by events in the operating theatre, the post-operative care must be such as to prevent patients dying from the effects of the original illness or of the operation itself.

The immediate aftercare of a patient who has undergone open-heart surgery is concerned with maintaining adequate circulation and ventilation, as the action of the heart and lungs has been disturbed. Vital functions such as arterial pressure, urine output, composition of blood gases and so on are constantly monitored until the patient's condition has fully stabilized. In the vast majority of cases the patient is conscious when taken from the operating theatre and returned to the intensive-care unit. The initial consideration must therefore be relief of pain, and this is achieved by injections of the strongest painkillers we have available – morphine or diamorphine (heroin). These opiate analgesics can cause respiratory depression and breathing problems, so that care must be taken when they are being used.

Haemorrhage is one of the main complications which we worry about in the days immediately after the operation. If it is external it is obvious, but internal bleeding cannot be seen; it can only be suspected if there is a rise in the pulse-rate and a fall in blood-pressure – this is why the post-operative nursing checks on the patient are so vital. If internal bleeding is suspected, the patient will need an immediate emergency operation to locate the source and stop the bleeding.

Within a few hours of the operation, passive massage of the legs is begun to prevent clot formation in the veins, and coughing exercises and chest physiotherapy are encouraged to prevent accretion of phlegm in the lungs. It is important that enough fluids are given to maintain the circulation volume and to keep the kidneys functioning adequately: this can be assessed by measuring the volume of urine passed and adjusting the amount of fluid given in the intravenous drip accordingly. Heart function is constantly reviewed by means of an electrocardiograph monitor at the bedside and, using a tube placed in the veins of the neck, by measuring the pressure of the large central veins where they enter the heart. Lung function is assessed by taking blood samples from an artery in the groin and measuring the concentration in them of gases, oxygen and carbon dioxide.

Patients often recuperate from major heart surgery a lot faster than from other operations such as removal of the gall bladder. Within a couple of days they will be out of bed, and they can expect to be discharged from hospital within 10 to 14 days. They are encouraged to increase their physical exercise gradually, so that by about 12 weeks after the operation they are fit, active and ready to enjoy all the things of life which have, for so long, been denied to them by their illness.

MECHANICAL HEARTS

Another answer to replacement hearts is to implant an artificial one. Think of the enormous advantages of such a heart – a machine of plastic and aluminium that, once implanted, could go on beating unrejected, permanently and reliably in

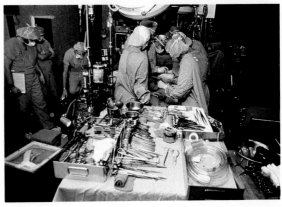

The artificial heart transplant in progress.

Barney Clark exercising after the operation.

the grateful chest of the recipient. Think, too, of Dr. Barney Clark who, on 2 December 1982, was given one such heart by Dr. William De Vries and his team at Utah University College of Medicine. Dr. Clark had developed a congestive cardiomyopathy and death was imminent. Two days after his artificial heart had been put in place the patient was talking to his doctors and his family, with healthily high blood-pressure. The world's first permanent artificial-heart patient seemed to be making a miraculous recovery.

Then things started to go wrong – lots of things. Barney had a series of seizures; part of the new heart had to be replaced; bubbles formed in his lungs – another operation; kidney failure; fits; a ten-day nose bleed... After 112 stormy post-operative days, Dr. Clark finally died. The 61-year-old patient's new heart, produced after 20 years of research and development, ultimately proved unequal to the task. And with his death the medical world began a massive appraisal, not only of the technical facility of mechanical hearts but of the desirability of pursuing this particular last resort.

There are, after all, huge problems and drawbacks. The patient has to be wired-up to a compressor which powers the heart, as no satisfactory compact internal or external power-source has yet been developed. Thus the quality of life for the patient is very much lower than it is for transplant survivors. However, experiments are continuing, and at the time of writing three more patients have been given artificial hearts.

When I carried out the first transplant operation the immediate reaction of many of my critics was, and still is, could not the vast sums of money needed to carry out further research be better spent elsewhere? Heart transplants are expensive operations and not always wondrous miracle cures. However, I do not think that this is any reason to spurn them. In the same way, neither should we turn our backs on the artificial heart as a concept unworthy of development. Things are improving all the time, and the day will surely come when engineers will be able to solve some of the as yet intractable problems. They will find a way of powering these man-made pumps, a technique for moving parts without

*Two views of the Jarvik-7 heart implanted
in Barney Clark. The major 'blood vessels' can
clearly be seen.*

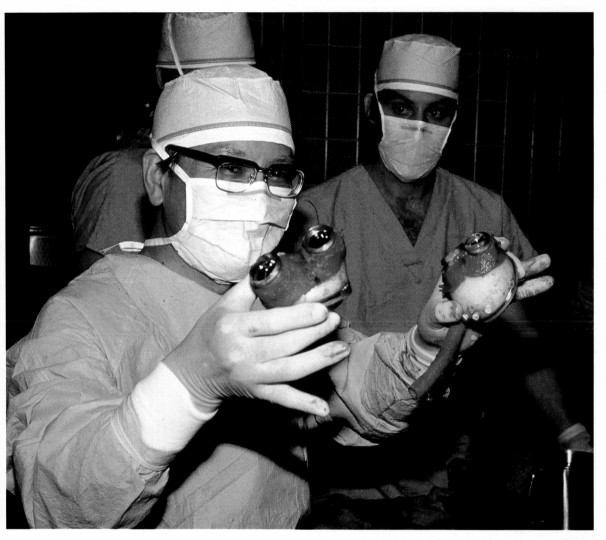

Other types of artificial heart are also being developed.

generating heat, a machine that fits in alongside a diseased organ and supplements rather than supplants its function. There is, I am sure, a future for the artificial heart although, even with improvements, I doubt whether it will take the place of biological transplants in the near future.

ARTIFICIAL PACEMAKERS

If, because of disease or ageing, the signal between the sinus node and the ventricles is interrupted, those all important pacing signals will fail to get through to maintain an adequate heartbeat (see Chapter 1). A slow heart leads to fatigue, breathlessness and the tell-tale symptom of swollen ankles, indicating oedema. Even more alarming, if the brain fails to get a supply of blood the outcome is giddiness, fainting and perhaps epileptic-type fits – even death.

Fortunately, within the past few years the drawbacks of a slow heartbeat have been overcome by the use of the pacemaker. This consists of a machine for generating pulses (the pacemaker itself), and an electrode lead or series of leads that take these signals to the ventricles, where they provide the necessary electrical stimulation. The pacing-box, with its associated wire or wires, is the electronic engineer's version of the sinus node.

The pacemaker itself is very light in weight, between 50 and 100 grams, and entirely enclosed in a fluid-tight casing. It derives its

A pacemaker.

power from a battery, usually a long-lasting lithium-type which can run for 10 years or so. (Early on, there were experiments with tiny nuclear-powered units and with rechargeable batteries, but these have been discarded on the ground of impracticability.) The currents generated by the power-pack are converted by electronic circuits into impulses. These travel down the electrode, which is really a kind of catheter through which run two insulated wires. At the heart end, these metal leads are exposed at the point where they enter the living tissue. Each impulse produced by the generator produces one heart-beat.

Nowadays the pace is geared to the demands of the body by a 'demand' pacemaker, which has replaced the out-of-date 'fixed-rate' pacemaker. Demand pacemakers, being sensitive to the natural beat of the heart, come into operation only when the heart misses its regular beats.

It is now possible to have programmable machines that can run either on demand or at a fixed rate, and the rate can also be adjusted, even though the device is actually implanted in the body. In fact, there have been some fascinating advances in pacemaker technology in recent years, especially in the marriage of electronic and biological materials. Scientists are busily developing microchips that will be responsive to living cells – 'biochips', to use the jargon – in order to make a device that will monitor very precisely certain chemical events

in the blood, especially adrenalin levels. In this way the pacemaker's output will exactly match the body's demands. Thus, as age or heart disease progressively slow down our heart-beat, the biochip will send to the pacemaker the appropriate instruction to speed up.

Implantation

Sometimes a slow heart-beat may develop in a person after a heart attack; in such cases, a pacemaker may be required to set the heart's pace for just a few days until the natural pump resumes normal operations. If so, the pacing-box can be strapped to the patient's arm and removed in a matter of seconds. More often, however, pacemakers need to be housed within the body for permanent deployment. This sounds a somewhat formidable undertaking, but in reality it is nothing of the sort.

The most widely used technique of implantation – the transvenous operation – is done under local anaesthetic and takes only about an hour. The pulse-generator is fitted between the skin and muscle of the chest and, being small, does not bulge out beyond the natural contours. The electrode lead is inserted in a vein in the shoulder or base of the neck and negotiated under X-ray scrutiny into the right ventricle of the heart.

Another type of implant is the epicardial implant, or 'epicardial' for short. Here the electrode lead is sewn onto the outer surface of the heart – the epicardium – while the pulse-generator box is housed in the abdominal wall.

Whatever the means of implanting used, the machine will be tested for proper functioning while the patient is still in hospital, and he or she will have an opportunity to discuss any questions of procedure, dos and don'ts, or anything else that comes to mind.

Check-ups over the telephone

Another development that is designed to ensure that the present generation of pacemaker-wearers do not run out of battery-power is the telephone check-up. Hitherto it has been necessary for a patient to make regular visits to the doctor for checks on the working condition of the machine: these checks involve quite sophisticated equipment, so they cannot be performed anywhere and everywhere. However, a small machine is now in use, principally in the USA, which will enable these checks to be carried out over the telephone.

The device is a box, the size of a packet of playing cards, that is rested on the chest. On top is a tiny loudspeaker against which the telephone mouthpiece is placed. The signals generated by the pacemaker are thus relayed down the telephone wire to a machine at the other end which analyses them and reports on the health of the pacemaker.

Telephone monitoring of pacemakers is not just a clever piece of medical maintenance work: it also helps dispel the worries that some people have about the effects of carrying a package of electronic instrumentation inside them. How, they may wonder, will their artificially aided heart perform if they walk too near to some electrical machine that might interfere with their pacemaker? This, I admit, can be a difficulty. Signals from electromagnets, spot-welding machines, metal detectors, anti-theft devices, television and radio transmitters, or even a faulty microwave oven could all, in theory, influence

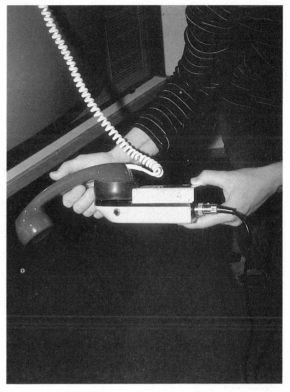

A telephone check-up.

the mechanisms of a pacemaker. But in practice interference signals are very rarely a problem. If you take proper care, I believe that there is absolutely no doubt that pacemakers, with all their enormous advantages, are preferable to no pacemaker and a slow-running heart.

A shock to the system

There is one further development in pacemaker technology that augurs well for those people at risk from potentially fatal abnormal heart-beats. Actually, the device is not really a pacemaker at all but a small compact version of the defibrillator used in hospitals for delivering heart-rousing electric shocks. Scientists have been testing a computer-controlled implantable defibrillator that delivers an electric current designed to restore normal heart-beat. So far 250 patients in 20 medical centres have been given these devices on the basis of their cardiac condition; to date the death-rate among them has been less than 5 percent. Without the machines, claim the researchers, the mortality from heart failure would have been around 60 percent.

An X-ray of a pacemaker implanted in the chest.

Chapter 5
Heart Attack and Counterattack

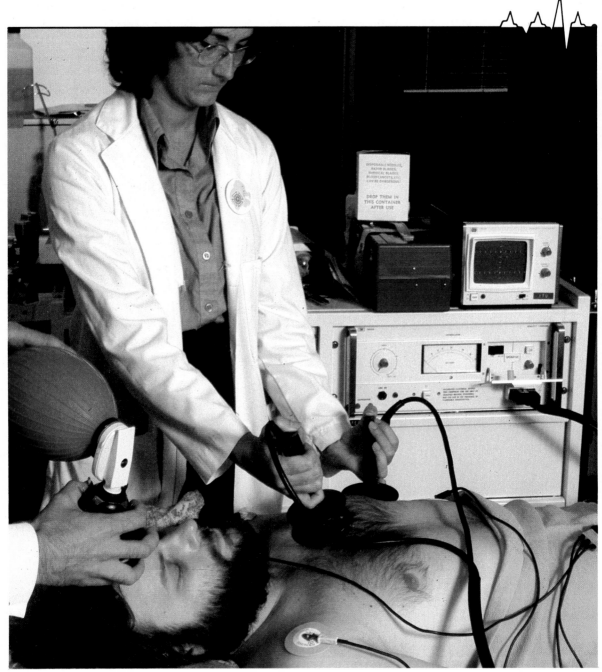

Before you reach the end of this paragraph someone, somewhere will have died from a heart attack. It will have happened apparently out of the blue, depriving the unsuspecting victim of life, often at the very peak of his or her existence. Up until now things were apparently fine, not a cloud in the sky, medically, emotionally or socially speaking. It could be your neighbour down the road, who has been doing so well in his or her small business. Your assistant, who always seems on top of things. Your spouse. Yourself?

Many doctors do not like the term 'heart attack'. They prefer to describe the sudden blockage of a coronary artery as 'coronary thrombosis' and the death of heart muscle as a 'myocardial infarction'. 'Infarct' is, for many of my colleagues, a better, more precise term than 'attack'. I do not agree. True, the medical terminology tells you more about the process of disease that causes the sudden onset of a heart in crisis. But 'attack' tells you far more about the vicious rapidity of it all. Moreover, the word suggests that there might be a *counter*attack; the assault on the citadel of the body might be repelled; or at least some post-attack measures to repair and restore might mitigate the effects.

For, mercifully, not all heart attacks are fatal. Indeed, the term 'heart attack' covers a wide range of experiences, from any sudden disturbance in the heart's function, such as a rhythm disorder, to a full-scale, lethal coronary heart attack. Even if the attack is not far short of fatal, there is still much that can be done. Your doctors will play their part but, in conjunction with the medical profession, patients and their families are vital, too. The whole task of coping with, recovering from and managing a heart attack is very definitely a collaborative business.

WHAT HAPPENS IN A HEART ATTACK?

The somewhat stereotyped picture of a heart attack to which we have grown accustomed in movies and television dramas is, perhaps surprisingly, close to the reality. First comes the tight crushing pain in the chest – angina – as the blood-supply to the heart begins to fail. Different patients have different ways of expressing the experience: 'Like having a heavy weight placed suddenly on the chest', according to one, while for another it is 'a tightening, a constriction like a giant clamp squeezing in on me'. Up to the critical moment people often feel perfectly well. When I talk to them afterwards it may transpire that, for the few days leading up to the attack, they had felt unduly tired, a bit short of breath, sometimes under a fair amount of pressure at work or perhaps some other stress at home. But they did not feel that these symptoms were going to trigger a heart attack. In fact, they tended to shrug off any warning signs as all part of everyday living.

Frightening pain

However, when this pain hits it is most definitely not like 'just' another angina attack, and it is too disturbing to be merely a bad attack of indigestion. The severe pain spreads from the chest to the neck and jaw regions. The face goes ashen, the lips and nails blue. Sitting down and taking a breather does not alleviate the symptoms, which are soon followed by heavy perspiration and feelings of faintness and nausea. It is an important signal that you need help. It is frightening and, as the attack subsides after a few hours, it leaves you feeling totally wiped out and exhausted. The emotional as well as the physical trauma is shattering. Angina is unlike other pain, and tends to induce a feeling of panic and fear of death which is unlike the response to other serious, even fatal, ailments.

ASSESSING ATTACK SEVERITY

What is the true nature of your attack? Is it mild and uncomplicated? Will you recover from it automatically without too much disturbance in your life? Or are you more seriously ill, needing intensive short-term care and careful long-term management, treatment by drugs or surgery, to enable you to survive? After the first attack, the road divides. Which route will you be taking?

Once any initial emergency measures have been taken, and the condition is stabilized, the patient is settled comfortably in bed and wired by electrodes to the ECG. At a glance, doctors and nurses can see on the screen a continuous visual picture of the heart's electrical activity. This is particularly vital for the first 24 hours or so after the attack, when sharp arrhythmias may mean that urgent medical intervention is necessary.

The patient stays in bed under close scrutiny while the severity of the condition is assessed and a course of treatment decided on. Step one is the interview, to elicit a detailed description of the attack: how the pain began, where it started and how it travelled; which parts of the body were affected, and so on. Good questioning and full answers are essential. The doctor will ask questions about any feeling of breathlessness on exertion or after meals. He will ask you to cast your mind back to any dizzy spells or faints you may have had. He will talk to you about any appointments you have made to visit a hospital in the past, for whatever reason, as well as your everyday state of health: appetite, weight, bowel and urine habits, menstrual patterns and irregularities, and so forth. And he will also talk about those factors we discussed earlier that make anyone a high-risk individual: smoking, previous high blood-pressure, high cholesterol levels, stress, and eating and drinking habits. If there is a family history of heart disease this will be noted.

There will also be a physical examination. Some of this will be good old-fashioned basic doctoring – pulse-rates, blood-pressure readings and so on. Some, though, will take you into the 'high-tech' environment of medical electronics and modern investigatory methods, all designed to give a sure diagnosis on which treatment can be based.

If your attack has been severe, you may already have come into contact with the 'hardware' of cardiology. Your heart may indeed have stopped altogether, and you may be alive still only because someone has acted quickly and you have been rushed into intensive care for electrical defibrillation; that massive shock (which you will not feel) to restart the passive heart. Or you may have already been put on a temporary pacemaker to keep your heart-rhythm up to normal speed.

EMERGENCY!

Heart attacks are no respecters of time, place or circumstance. While some victims manage to walk into their doctor's surgery or casualty department complaining of a 'bit of a pain in the chest', it is a daunting statistic that one in every two heart-attack deaths occur within a couple of hours unless assistance is at hand; it is here that you, the bystander, can help. Research in the United States has shown that, where bystanders have been trained in resuscitation techniques, the likelihood of a heart attack being fatal is significantly reduced. So what should you do?

If the patient is conscious, telephone their doctor or call an ambulance, explaining that you think the person has had a heart attack. If he or she is unconscious, get someone to call an ambulance while you check the pulse, either at

A specially trained cardiac ambulance team in action. First oxygen, mechanical ventilation and cardiac massage, but the heart is still not beating! The portable defibrillator is used to restart the heart. Drugs are administered intravenously to counteract shock. Finally the victim can be moved into the ambulance.

the neck or on the chest below the left nipple. If no pulse can be felt you have approximately three minutes to do something – so don't waste time looking for dilated pupils or checking the breathing. With your fist, strike as hard a blow as you can over the lower part of the breast-bone. On occasion this may be enough to start the heart again; but, if within 15 to 20 seconds it hasn't, then start cardio-pulmonary resuscitation.

The principles behind this procedure are really quite simple. The heart-attack victim needs air and circulating blood and these are what you are providing. Check that there is nothing blocking the mouth (false teeth and vomit are the main culprits) and then tilt the head right back to straighten the windpipe. Pinch the victim's nose, cover his or her mouth with yours and blow slowly but firmly into the mouth. You should notice the chest going up and down as the air

enters the patient's lungs. If not, the patient has a blockage, so check the mouth again. Blow into the lungs three or four times.

Now either you or a helper should kneel on the right side of the patient (the opposite side if you are left-handed), put the heel of your left hand on the lower third of the victim's breast-bone, cover it with your right hand and rock forward and backward, squeezing the chest as you go. What you are doing now is simply squeezing the heart between the breast-bone and the back-bone, and thereby pushing the blood out into the circulation. When you rock back the heart expands, sucking in blood ready for you to squeeze out again when you rock forward. By alternating ten heart contractions to three or four breaths into the lungs, you can keep the patient alive for 20 to 30 minutes, or even longer, by which stage the ambulance should have arrived.

The ambulancemen will put a plastic airway into the patient's mouth, and through this they will give oxygen while they continue resuscitation until they reach hospital.

The resuscitation team will have been summoned and will be waiting at casualty; this team consists of a group of doctors and nurses each with a specific job to do in the event of a patient collapsing after a heart attack. Following impairment of the circulation, acids which can be toxic collect in the bloodstream and tissues. An intravenous drip will be put in the arm and, through this, small quantities of sodium bicarbonate will be given to neutralize the acid. At the same time another doctor will place an

First Aid

If the victim is not breathing, start mouth-to-mouth resuscitation (Kiss of Life) immediately.

1   Quickly clear the mouth of any dirt or vomit, etc.

2   Bend the head backwards with one hand and push the jaw upwards with the other hand. This lifts the tongue off the back of the throat. This action alone may allow breathing to start.

3   If not, quickly give the victim 4 full breaths: Pinch the nostrils together then take a deep breath in, seal your lips around the mouth and blow into it. See that the chest rises as you blow in.

4   Take your mouth away and watch the chest fall.

5   After 4 full breaths, check the pulse to see if the heart is beating. Can you feel the carotid pulse? Put two fingers into the groove at the side of the victim's Adam's apple and press firmly. If you can feel a pulse, continue mouth-to-mouth resuscitation giving 16 to 18 breaths per minute (one every 3 to 4 seconds) until breathing starts again.

If you can't feel a pulse, and the victim's face is ashen or purple, the heart has stopped beating: start heart resuscitation. (Never attempt heart resuscitation if the heart is beating.)

1   Lie the victim on his back on the floor or other firm surface, and kneel alongside.

2   Put the heel of one hand on the lower half of the breast bone, and cover it with the heel of the other hand. Press down hard on the lower half of the breast bone to a depth of about 1½ inches. Press

about 80 times a minute. To help you keep time, count out a rhythm of 'one and ... two and ... three and ...' as you do it.

3 The victim will not start breathing again until the heart has started beating. So after pressing 15 times, stop the heart resuscitation and give 2 quick breaths by mouth-to-mouth resuscitation as described.

Continue to give 15 presses and 2 breaths in this way.

If there is another person with you, get them to do the heart resuscitation. Give 5 presses, 1 breath, 5 presses, 1 breath, without pausing. Press about 60 times a minute. To help you keep time, count out a rhythm of 'one thousand and one ... one thousand and two ... one thousand and three ...' as you do it.

4 After one minute, check the carotid pulse to see if the heart has restarted. Then keep checking every three minutes, or until the colour of the face begins to improve.

Continue heart resuscitation until the heart starts beating.

5 Once the heart has started beating keep on with mouth-to-mouth resuscitation until breathing starts again.

6 Once the breathing has started, put the person into the recovery position (lying on his side with the head to one side so that the tongue does not block the airway). Wait for medical help to arrive.

7 Stay with the person, watching all the time in case the breathing or heart stop again.

endotracheal tube through the mouth down into the lungs, so that oxygen can be given directly.

Most deaths from heart attacks are due to ventricular fibrillation. In this condition the heart-muscle, instead of contracting in an orderly fashion, contracts frequently and randomly. The resulting quivering (so that the heart is rather aptly described as looking like a bag of wriggling worms) is of insufficient force to pump blood around the body. To counteract this, the technique of electrical defibrillation is used. Two paddles, each about the size of a beermat,

The equipment available in a cardiac ambulance.

are placed on the chest, one on either side of the heart. A short, sharp electric current (200-400 joules) is passed from one paddle to the other through the heart. This is often sufficient to literally 'shock' the heart out of its abnormal behaviour and back into a regular rhythm.

With the heart beating again, the patient is brought to the coronary care unit. This is the 'hi-tech' part of the hospital which usually amazes and dismays visitors who come to see their loved ones, only to find them wired up to complex machines and with tubes visible just about everywhere. Let me try and simplify it.

If the patient is unconscious and breathing

A defibrillator.

badly he or she may need assistance to breathe, and so will need to have an endotracheal tube attached to a mechanical ventilator, which takes over the job of breathing for the patient. Electrodes attached to the chest will run to a monitor (like a television screen) beside the bed and another in the nurses' station. This allows the patient's heart-rate and rhythm to be

An intensive care unit's central monitoring station, Dallas, Texas.

checked and, most importantly, may give warning of complications so that they may be prevented. Intravenous drip-lines are run into the arm, and through these fluids, drugs and food, if necessary, are given. Another intravenous tube will probably be placed in a vein in the neck to measure central venous pressure, an important indicator of how well the heart is pumping. Finally, a catheter is placed in the bladder through which urine can drain into a bag at the side of the bed.

The whole purpose of the coronary care unit is to predict, prevent or, if that is not possible, to treat quickly any complications of the heart attack. The most likely of these complications is an abnormal rhythm, fast and/or irregular, for which an anti-arrhythmic drug such as lignocaine, desopyramide or procainamide is given, or a slowing of the heart, for which atropine may be administered. Certain types of heart attack can affect the conducting system of the heart, so that the atria and ventricles contract at different rates. When a complete heart block (as this is called) occurs the heart may beat too slowly to be

A close-up of some of the emergency equipment, showing an arrhythmia computer and oscilloscope.

efficient, and therefore an electrical pacemaker may be inserted into the heart through a vein, and the heart thereby stimulated to beat more rapidly. Failure of the heart to pump adequately can sometimes lead to fluid collecting in the lungs or abdomen, and drugs may be used so that this excess fluid is removed and excreted in the urine.

The last two decades have seen a dramatic reduction in the period of bed-rest recommended after a heart attack. If the attack is not complicated by an abnormal rhythm or heart failure, the patient will normally be out of bed in a few days and discharged home within a week or ten days. The area of heart-muscle affected by the heart attack will take four to six weeks to be replaced with scar tissue, and so during this time it is probably wise to restrict vigorous activities; physical activities can then gradually be increased, with the prospect of returning to work and a normal lifestyle within three months of the original heart attack. This timetable obviously has to be adjusted for those with complications or an exceptionally heavy or stressful job. Throughout every stage, encouragement and reassurance should be forthcoming from doctors, friends and relatives, since more people are incapacitated by the psychological aftermath of a heart attack than by the actual physical effects.

A patient in a coronary care unit. He is fitted with a temporary external pacemaker, drip and oxygen mask.

POST-ATTACK: WHAT NEXT?

What a wonderfully resilient organ the heart is. The majority of people who have a heart attack will recover from the experience and, once the initial phase of acute illness is over, will return home from hospital to lead a normal – or, at worst, near-normal – life. As for the unfortunate minority of really serious cases, their existence will certainly be impaired, but even for them, given the benefits of powerful heart drugs taken long-term, or of surgery, the outlook is not totally bleak – in fact, it is very good.

Exercise tests may well be performed on patients, just before they leave the hospital (between the twelfth and fourteenth day) and/or before they return to work (around six to eight weeks after the attack). Those patients whose

A heart patient undergoing post-operative care in hospital.

capacity for effort seems abnormally low and who have an abnormal blood-pressure response (particularly if there is recurrent angina and the serial ECGs during the exercise tests document evidence of ischemia) will be given a coronary arteriogram. This is to check on whether the patient has disease in vessels other than those which have shown a blockage at the time of the attack. In other words, it is a test not only of the recovery of heart muscle following the attack but also of future damage to the remaining heart muscle which might be caused by previously undetected disease in the coronary vessels. Work in this area is relatively recent, and there is a large European trial in progress called 'The Survivors Trial', studying the best management of those patients who show abnormal results in exercise tests soon after a heart attack. Some patients are being put forward for coronary-artery graft procedures, others are being

It will take a while to return to normal after a heart attack, so it helps to find a relaxing activity.

managed with optimum medical measures, but all receive advice regarding prevention (no smoking, dietary improvement, weight control, and so on.

The exercise test performed between four and 10 weeks after a heart attack may find an established role, not only in assessing the level of recovery and any residual coronary disease, but also in showing the patient the levels of activity that he or she can safely perform on returning to daily life. A good response from the exercise test is most reassuring for the patient, who can then virtually forget his or her heart attack and concentrate fully on a normal life, having learnt how to avoid the risk factors that precipitated the first (and, with luck, only) heart attack.

The average heart-attack patient will, after leaving hospital, almost always feel a bit anxious, shaken up by the events of the past few days or weeks and a little fearful of what this all implies for everyday living. He or she will also feel the weakness and slight depression one gets after, say, a heavy bout of influenza. All this is perfectly normal and natural, and it should not blind one to the fact that, within a few months or so after the attack, strength will return and with it the confidence to get back into a normal routine.

Take it easy

Constant contact with your doctor is essential. He will give you hints and advice on how to build up strength without overdoing things, and give you advice about sensible habits, such as short afternoon naps during convalescence and early nights as a general rule. You may not be able to progress as rapidly as you feel you should – or would like. Indeed, you may get frustrated and try to hurry things along by overexertion – frenzied spells to catch up on the gardening or housework, and so on. Or you may be comparing your own progress with that of a friend or relative who has also had an attack and who – at the same stage as you now are – seemed to be doing so much more.

I understand these feelings and have many times seen them in action, driving patients to levels of activity that are quite inappropriate for their current capabilities. But people vary very widely in every aspect of health: one person's gentle stroll is another's agonizing marathon. So remember, exercise within your own limits and never try to force the pace. Talk about your progress with your doctor who, as a result of skilful questioning, will be able to tell you how far you can comfortably and safely go. Never try to *drive* yourself into health. Recovering from a major event such as a heart attack or a bypass operation must be a gradual, cumulative process. Every day you will feel a little better and will be able to take on a little more: a second turn around the block with the dog; a few more lengths of the swimming bath; a gentle outing on your bicycle.

In fact, I find that physical exercise regimes are not usually much of a problem during these early days. Rather more worrying for many is the mental strain and emptiness of being away from work, restricted in what they can do, and still anxious about the future. If you are a heart-attack patient or have one close to you, make an extra effort in this direction. Look for mental stimulation, taking up or perhaps reviving an abandoned hobby, listening to more music, reading more, catching up on that unanswered correspondence.

Make sure you are absolutely ready before you do more physical exertion during the recovery period.

Occupy yourself

Having advised you to take things easy after an attack, I want now to flip the coin and warn you not to coddle yourself into becoming an over-sensitive body likely to crack at the slightest interference or stress. Up until the 1950s doctors used to counsel prolonged bed-rest for heart patients, but this did not work very well. You cannot immobilize the heart the way you might a broken bone in plaster. The big disadvantage of confining a person to bed is that it tends to throw the patient into a solitary state of anxiety and invalidity. Prostrate and lonely,

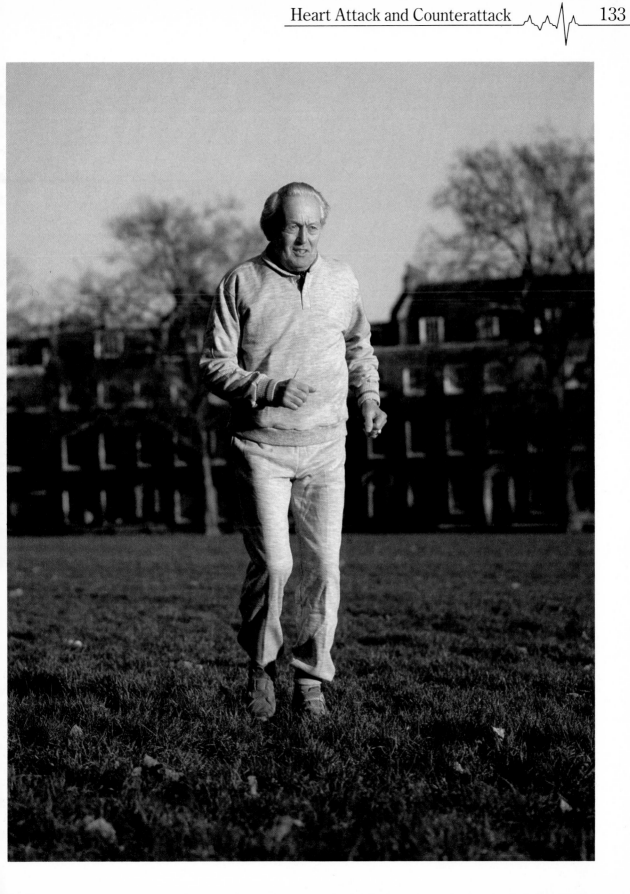

the convalescent patient is constantly bearing out those lines from *Hamlet:* 'There is nothing either good or bad, but thinking makes it so.' And, generally, thinking about illness makes it worse. Better to be up and about.

GETTING BACK TO NORMAL

There are some people – perhaps everyone to a greater or lesser degree – who for a while after a heart attack gradually enjoy their new condition of 'heart victim'; what one researcher into

Reform of dietary habits is essential after a heart attack.

people's reactions to illness, Dr. Una Maclean, once described as 'the benefits of martyrdom'. But after a very short while this fails to console the recoverer. What most people want to know most urgently is: 'When can I go back to work?'

As you might expect, I am reluctant to give anyone too specific an answer to this most crucial question. So much will depend on progress in the early post-attack period. As a matter of fact, most people are back at work within a few weeks, although obviously the more severe the attack and the more demanding the job, both physically and emotionally, the longer one must expect to wait. However, employers are

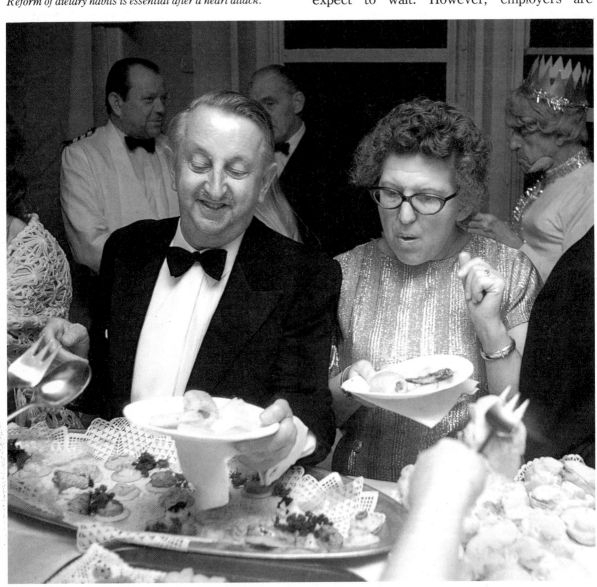

increasingly aware that they can help in the recuperation process by offering lighter work or part-time hours to begin with. The key indicator of fitness is your performance in the exercise tests, which must be interpreted by an expert, but there are also some general guidelines to help you and your doctor decide on whether you are fit to return to the occupational fray:

Are you feeling confident about your ability to manage things? If so, you are probably not far off starting.

Can you take a briskish walk for a couple of kilometres without getting distressed? If so, you can take on most non-manual work.

How much stress will be involved in returning to work? If you are going to face a very taxing work environment, with lots of haste and bustle, don't take the step too quickly. In fact, while you are off work think about getting another job. Stress is a potential killer.

Is your job one of those, such as airline pilot or train driver, where a recurrence of heart trouble could have catastrophic effects not just for you but for hundreds of others as well? If so, there are probably regulations barring you from returning to the same job. Even if there are not, think carefully, in consultation with your doctor, before throwing yourself back into a high-risk job.

Is sex dangerous?
When people ask me this question, which they do very frequently, I am inclined to answer: 'Only if you don't indulge in it.' Stories are legion about men who have had a fatal coronary while in the very act of having intercourse (usually during adultery!), but these are apocryphal. Having intercourse involves physical exertion, it is true, but this is not much more than that needed to walk up two flights of stairs. So if you have made it upstairs to the bedroom without discomfort you can confidently enjoy yourself therein.

Should you find that sex makes you abnormally breathless or, on occasions, gives you a twinge of angina, then do not immediately retreat into invalidity and stop altogether. Relax. Slow down. Change your immediate method of lovemaking

for something a bit more languid. It does not have to be full of sound and fury to be highly enjoyable. Use care and imagination instead of acrobatics. You will not be disappointed.

Both men and women may experience a reduction in their sexual urges after a heart attack, and men may have trouble getting an erection. But this is usually due to the fear, lassitude and depression that one might experience at this time: if sex becomes a difficulty in the wake of an infarct, this is usually because of a problem of attitude rather than of bodily function. After all, the most important sexual organ is, as the cliché has it, the brain.

What about driving?
Long hours behind the wheel of a heavy truck may never again be possible, but the normal domestic and business use of an automobile is often perfectly acceptable after two or three months, although rarely before. After 10 weeks or so you can tell whether sudden angina attacks are likely to recur, and if they do, wait a while before you think of getting back behind the wheel. Even if you feel 'well enough' to drive, ask yourself how you respond to cutting your way through the traffic jungle. Are you the type who takes it all calmly, or do you react badly? If you are the finger-tapping, quick-tempered, aggressive type of driver, then do not be in a hurry to use the car again.

What changes will I have to make in my lifestyle?
If the attack patient is, say, a professional athlete who is faced with immediate loss of his or her combined livelihood and absorbing passion, of course painful changes will have to be made. It is sometimes a life-or-death decision, and most people opt for life, however second-best this at first appears. But such tragic dilemmas are comparatively rare. More often, the fact that a person has had a heart attack makes that individual more aware of how precious life is and what can be done to preserve and enhance it.

For example, people ask about food. Will they be confined to a restricted range of 'heart' diets for the rest of their days? The answer is 'no'. What attack victims must do is eat less fatty food, keep down their weight, stop smoking and prefer an active to a sedentary existence. Does that sound 'special'? To me this seems merely an obvious formula for living a longer, healthier life.

What sort of help can I get?

Here of course the first port of call with any problems and worries must be your doctor. Increasingly, however, self-help groups for heart-attack patients and their partners are beginning to spring up. These provide a meeting point for people to share their experiences and anxieties, a place to swap stories and ideas about rehabilitation and how it can be speeded along. Some groups organize guest speakers and advisers, such as trained nurses, to give practical advice on topics such as choosing effort-saving devices for the home. Such clubs are very useful in helping you find understanding with people who are going or have been through the same mill as you.

Will I have another attack?

The after-effects of a heart attack differ from case to case: a minority of people have no problems at all, but the majority suffer recurrent problems such as breathlessness due to heart-muscle or valve damage, or recurrent angina and the risk of another heart attack. The complex of risk factors which contributed to the first attack will, unless altered for the better, determine the likelihood of a second one occurring. About some of these risk factors, such as a family history of coronary-artery disease, nothing can be done, but others can be reduced. Measures such as losing weight if you are obese, increasing exercise if you are sedentary, reducing the saturated-fat intake in your diet, controlling blood-fat levels (if you are a younger patient) and, most importantly of all, stopping cigarette-smoking can, to varying degrees, reduce your risk of a subsequent heart attack. Most victims interpret their attack as a warning to alter their lifestyle and therefore do take steps to reduce the chances of a recurrence.

Many people who have had a heart attack, even with ventricular fibrillation requiring resuscitation, do very well and survive into old age. One in two sufferers will live for 10 years after their attack and one in every four will survive for 20 years or more – figures which compare very favourably with many of the other diseases and afflictions which may befall us.

These facts should be reassuring to someone who has had a heart attack. It is not the end of the world. True, some changes may have to be made to your lifestyle, but the likelihood is that you will live for many happy and trouble-free years.

PREVENTION AS COUNTERATTACK: COMBATING HYPERTENSION

Whatever results you may have derived for yourself from the risk-factor chart, there is no need to be a passive recipient of what fate may have in store for you by way of a second attack. Remember my version of CHD: Care Helps Deter. This is just as true for the person recovering from a heart attack and anxious to avoid another as it is for someone who has never had the slightest indication that he or she has coronary heart disease. Part II of this book gives you a complete programme to keep the heart healthy; but before you get to that I want to go into some detail about the causes and treatments of high blood-pressure.

Of all the factors that are thought to lead to heart disease, there is one about which I have no doubts at all: high blood-pressure, commonly known as hypertension. It is undeniably a public enemy, being responsible not only for cardiac disorders but also for some cases of kidney failure and strokes. It becomes a stronger risk factor the older one gets, and it is as detrimental to women as it is to men.

Consider these chilling facts:

Hypertension is the commonest chronic disease in the USA, affecting 35 million people with a further 25 million on the borderline.

In the USA hypertension is thought to cause around 500 000 cases of stroke each year – and, of these, 175 000 deaths.

Hypertension is implicated in the 1 250 000 heart attacks that occur each year in the USA.

People whose blood-pressure is in the top 20 percent of the total range are twice as likely to succumb to coronary heart disease as the 20 percent at the bottom.

In order to maintain a supply of blood to all parts of our body, the heart has to pump fluid at a certain pressure, just as the water-supply in your home is circulated under pressure to the various taps and other outlets. Even in healthy individuals, blood-pressure varies quite a lot during the day to meet the differing demands of the body: the greater the physical and psychological stresses, the higher our blood-pressure rises, while, as we sleep, it drops to its lowest levels. Springing out of bed in the morning activates the automatic regulatory mechanism to raise the pressure. You may have noticed that sometimes the response of this mechanism is a bit sluggish, so that when you sit or stand up suddenly from a resting position you feel light-headed or dizzy. This is because the pressure has not yet reached a point where it is sufficient to send an adequate supply of blood to the brain, so there is a brief blood drought.

Regulating the blood supply

There is a feedback mechanism to ensure that supply and demand are kept in harmony. This works by routing information on how much blood is needed to the appropriate centre in the brain, which in turn initiates the production of 'stress hormones' such as adrenalin. These galvanize the system into activity, stimulating the heart to pump more powerfully and at the same time constricting the blood vessels slightly: more volume of blood passing through a smaller-circumference tube leads to increased pressure. When the appropriate level is reached, the information that this is so is fed back to the brain, which decreases the adrenalin output. The pressure is eased off the throttle and the body-machine slows down.

The feedback mechanism controlling blood pressure.

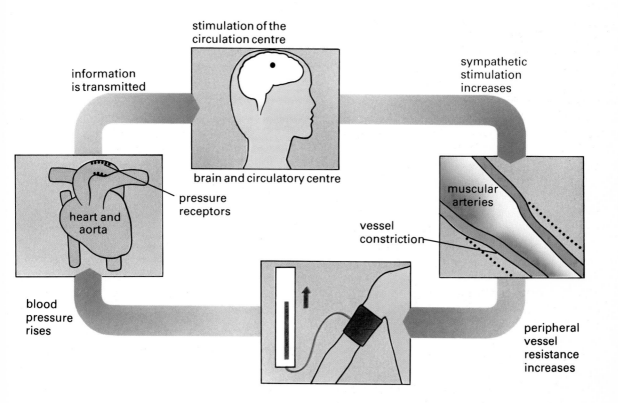

Too high is dangerous

It is quite common for, say, a man aged 35 to 40 to be technically hypertensive without any complicating symptoms: no headaches, dizzy spells or bouts of hot flushes. It is only five, ten or even more years later that a symptom does present itself, and when it does it can be dramatic: the overworked heart can fail, or the extra pressure in the blood vessels can result in a stroke.

In the long term, hypertension damages the linings of the arteries. Instead of flowing smoothly and evenly, the blood is crashing and buffeting along against the arterial walls like flood waters in a cellar. At points of maximum turbulence, small patchy deposits of diseased tissue may form – atheroma – or the arteries may harden – atherosclerosis – causing some impairment in blood flow or even total blockage. The heart is deprived of nourishment while at the same time the fatigued heart muscle is being forced to pump against increased arterial resistance. Unless something is done, a heart attack could be just around the corner.

Measuring blood-pressure

One way to reduce the chances of becoming one of the millions who fall victim to the complications caused by hypertension is by keeping a regular watch on your blood-pressure levels. The procedure is quick, painless and instructive. If you are in your mid-thirties or over, you should make sure that your blood-pressure is checked once a year.

A routine blood-pressure reading is usually taken while you are sitting in a relaxed position. One of the instruments used to measure blood pressure is the sphygmomanometer – sphygmo, for short – which is usually nothing more than a mercury pressure-gauge attached to a cuff which fits around your upper arm. Once in place this cuff is inflated to block off the pulse at the elbow, the idea here being to obtain a reading independent of the peaks and troughs of the pulse. Then a stethoscope is placed over the main arm artery, and the air in the cuff is released through a valve, thereby allowing the jammed-up blood to rush through again. As it does so, a sound is heard in the stethoscope earpiece which is characteristic of the upper, or systolic, blood-pressure. This is recorded on the mercury tube or dial. Then, as the blood continues to flow through the artery, the cuff is further deflated and the sound of the now evenly flowing blood suddenly fades away – this is the point at which the reading for the lower, or diastolic, pressure is recorded.

So, measuring air-pressures, what the sphygmo does is tell you the amount of pressure exerted on the walls of the artery by blood from

Taking blood pressure readings.

Horsing around at the Royal Society

The modern sphygmomanometer – a familiar sight in every general practitioner's office – was foreshadowed by the curious experiments of a parish priest named Stephen Hales, who, in the eighteenth century, inserted a brass tube into an artery in a horse's neck. To this pipe he attached a glass tube and watched in fascination as the blood from this equine collaborator rose up above heart level to a height of 8 feet 3 inches (2.51 m). Not unnaturally, the horse grew restless at being used as a medical guinea-pig, and her pulse rate increased. The level in the glass rose and fell in time with the pulse, suggesting that the process of measuring blood-pressure could be truly accurate only if done while the pulse was temporarily obliterated. So, while brass tubes inserted into arteries did not emerge as the regular method of taking pressures, Hales' investigations (which he later recounted to the prestigious Royal Society in London) did establish both the principle of the sphygmo and the need to eliminate the pulse fluctuations.

the heart (the systolic pressure) and the amount to which the pressure drops while the heart is refilling (the diastolic pressure). It is a simple and reliable device for most purposes. Only when extreme accuracy is needed does a doctor resort to a more sophisticated technique involving a tube inserted directly into the artery.

What readings constitute 'normal'? This varies with age; the levels given here, measured in mmHg or 'millimetres of mercury' are used by doctors as a guide. For young adults the 'normotensive' readings are: systolic – under

140 mmHg; diastolic – under 90 mmHg. This is written as 140/90. The normotensive readings for elderly males are 160/100 and for elderly females 170/90.

Young adults who have a systolic reading of between 140 and 159 and a diastolic reading between 90 and 94 would be categorized as 'borderline hypertensive', and if the systolic reading is above 160 and the diastolic above 95, this indicates 'significant hypertension'.

Actually, readings can sometimes be misleading. I have known doctors use battered old sphygmos that look as if they had been picked up secondhand 25 years ago, and which probably give inaccurate readings. An undersized cuff can record a falsely high pressure – a potential problem if your arms are on the fat side. Do not hesitate, therefore, either to question a reading that surprises you, or indeed to seek a second opinion from a doctor whom you know to have updated this equipment.

WHAT CAUSES HYPERTENSION?

For about 15 percent of hypertensives the underlying cause can often be identified. These cases of 'secondary' hypertension may be provoked by a specific defect in the mechanisms that regulate blood-flow. For example, a narrowing of the arteries will reduce blood-supply to the kidneys and thereby increase blood-pressure. Other types of constriction, kidney disorder, hormonal abnormality and, on rare occasions, tumours will all increase blood-pressure to hypertensive levels. But these identifiable disorders account for only a small minority of hypertension sufferers.

The lion's share of hypertensives, 85 percent, are so-called 'essential' or 'primary' hypertensives, who must look to other causes. And now we are moving into the realm of informed guesswork, because primary hypertension is still something of a mystery, and in assessing it we have to rely on clues rather than on incontrovertible evidence.

Heredity
Primary hypertension tends to run in families, and racial factors are also important. For instance, a greater percentage of US blacks suffer from high blood-pressure than do US whites. However, families and, to a lesser extent, racial groups within a single country or area do tend to follow roughly the same lifestyle, eat the same food and so on, so it may be that some causes attributed to 'nature' may in fact have their origins in 'nurture'. And, even if they do not, it is to the environmental factors that we are forced to turn next: you can, after all, do something about your lifestyles, whereas you cannot choose your parents.

Dietary factors and weight
If your weight is 20 percent above the norm for your height and frame, you are three times as likely to develop high blood-pressure than is a person of average weight for the same height and frame. Going on a reducing diet therefore seems an obvious first step for anyone who is overweight and has high-blood pressure.

Another factor closely associated with hypertension is our intake of salt. To ensure health we need to take in about 4 grams of salt (sodium chloride) a day, but it is quite normal for us to consume daily two, three or even more times that amount. It now seems clear that this excess sodium consumption is positively injurious. Somehow (the exact mechanism is not known) salt affects the walls of the arteries and changes their sensitivity to stimulation.

One problem for those who might wish to reduce the amount of salt they eat is that of being able to find out where the enemy lurks. Even if you stop adding salt to food while cooking or eating it, this removes only part of the danger. Two-thirds of our salt intake comes by way of processed foods, to which salt has already been added. In order to cut down salt effectively we must either do without processed foods altogether or buy the special low-salt products which are now becoming more widely available. You should also watch out for certain pharmaceutical products which contain sodium, especially ones designed to treat hangovers and stomach disorders. Examine carefully the labels on anything you buy for sodium content.

But probably the biggest stumbling block for most adults is simply that they *like* salty foods; their palates have become conditioned to them. If that is the case, cut down gradually on salt, and try using herbs and spices instead.

Smoking, drinking and stress

Less pronounced but nevertheless detectable is the relationship between alcohol and cigarette consumption and high blood-pressure. Now here, as with salt, I do not advocate an immediate and drastic cessation of all such activity. However, if you refer to the sections on alcohol (Chapter 9) and smoking (Chapter 8), you will see how you can cut down.

You should refer also to my strategies for combating stress (Chapter 7), because too much tension and anxiety are associated with hypertension. Also, stress certainly has short-term effects on blood-pressure, because it galvanizes the nervous and hormonal systems into surges of hyperactivity.

SYMPTOMS OF HYPERTENSION

Hypertension is a 'silent killer'. People suffering from this serious health hazard may display no

Obesity contributes to high blood pressure.

symptoms, the only sign being a 'high' reading on the sphygmo if they have a check-up. On the other hand, some people may experience such symptoms as nervousness, palpitations, dizziness, chest pain, headaches and a general feeling of mental lassitude or depression – maybe not all of these symptoms, perhaps just one or two. The trouble is, of course, that these non-specific signals could be indicative of quite a few other complaints as well: they can arise because of constipation, bronchitis, hangover or whatever. Indeed, the danger is that you are half-inclined to put them down to being not as young as you were, or invoke some other bland explanation. All the while, though, the hypertension is there, damaging your arterial circulation, putting stress on a heart that is finding it more and more difficult to cope.

This all makes it difficult to know what is going on – until, of course, at last there is a rapid deterioration and you succumb to heart disease. However, if you want to be ahead of the game and be alert to hypertension before complications set in, get your pressure checked once a year. If you have any of the symptoms listed below, get a check-up immediately, as these are signs that hypertension might be causing damage.

Shortness of breath after the minimum of exertion, especially if there is a persistent cough.

Swelling of the ankles (oedema), especially if this persists throughout the day.

Chest pains and/or tightness in chest, perhaps radiating towards the neck, left shoulder, left arm and hand.

Dizziness and memory lapses, any speech problems, weakness in arms and legs and walking difficulties; leg cramp making it difficult to move about without frequent rests.

Any other signs, such as excessive sweating, anxiety and discomfort, including vague feelings in the region of the heart which worry you.

If the doctor diagnoses hypertension, a variety of treatments are possible, each tailored to individual needs. Fortunately, this is one of those exciting areas in medicine where considerable strides have been taken in recent years, so, if you have acted early enough, the outlook is promising.

Sometimes a doctor will recommend that the hypertensive initially tries to control blood-pressure levels by a few changes in lifestyle, concerning smoking, weight, diet, exercise and so on, as changing to a more healthy daily regime may be preferable to undertaking a course of drugs. What is more, quite a few cases of hypertension remit spontaneously: in the course of time, pressure levels can fall and thereafter remain within the normal bracket, so that the disease simply goes away.

In other cases, and in more serious circumstances, doctors will have recourse to some of the remarkable anti-hypertension drugs now available. Once the pressure has been reduced to the right level, the aim is to maintain this without introducing some of the side-effects that these drugs can cause, such as feeling faint on sitting or standing, diarrhoea, mood changes, blurred vision, drowsiness and, sometimes, changes in sexual urge or function.

DRUGS USED IN TREATING HYPERTENSION

Diuretics

Beta blockers and diuretics (described in detail in Chapter 4) are both used to control hypertension. In addition a variety of other drugs are effective. The oldest are the *rauwolfia* compounds and their derivatives, used for centuries as sedatives, which act by eliminating some of the noradrenalin stored in the walls of the arteries and thereby reducing the action of the hormone on the tissues and nerves. The *methyldopa* group of drugs also reduce tension-provoking adrenalin, this time by tricking the body into producing a harmless,

Oedema is a common symptom of hypertension.

Hypertension: a prevention checklist

1 Control your weight. If you need to lose 10 to 20 kg, do it. And try to keep your weight there.

2 Go easy on the salt! Don't add salt to food before or after cooking. As far as possible avoid processed foods.

3 Watch smoking and alcohol levels. Preferably, stop the former altogether and restrict the latter to one or two drinks a day (one drink being a glass of wine, a small scotch, a half-pint of beer, or the equivalent).

4 Exercise regularly.

5 Have regular blood-pressure checks as recommended by your doctor.

6 If you are on tablets, follow the prescribed doses. An expert on hypertension therapy believes that as many as four-fifths of patients fail to stick to what their doctors recommend.

7 Learn some simple de-stressing techniques, as described in Chapter 7, especially to enable you to get a good night's sleep.

8 Try to take at least one holiday from work each year.

---

non-stimulating chemical instead. *Clonidine* has a more direct action on the central nervous system, producing a sedative effect on the individual and so reducing both heart-rate and blood-pressure. Among the most powerful of all anti-hypertensive agents are the group including *guanethidine*. These act to block the transmission of electrochemical messages from the brain to blood vessels, shutting off the impulses in the nerves that supply arteries and in so doing lowering the resistance of those arteries to blood flowing through them.

Anti-hypertensive drugs

There are two other new anti-hypertensive drug groups, *calcium blockers* and *angiotensin-converting enzyme inhibitors*.

The calcium blockers dilate peripheral arterial walls by preventing calcium from exerting its contracting effect on the constricting circular muscles of the arterial wall. Vasodilation, as the effect is called, increases the calibre of the run-off blood vessels and therefore lowers the pressure required to fill them. This group of drugs is useful for lowering all grades of hypertension, but is particularly efficacious for treating a raised diastolic pressure and for patients with associated kidney disease. Calcium blockers combine well with beta blockers to assist patients who also have an adrenalin-

related rise in their established hypertension.

Angiotensin-converting enzyme inhibitors are very useful for the treatment of cases of hypertension that will not respond to other treatment, particularly if the hypertension has been complicated by heart failure (shortness of breath and fluid accumulation). To treat hypertension, your doctor will choose initially a diuretic, a beta blocker or a calcium blocker. He or she will probably then go on to combine two or all three of these to gain appropriate control of the blood-pressure under all circumstances (resting, standing, and after mild exertion such as walking up a flight of stairs). If, despite these measures, the blood-pressure still remains uncontrolled, the doctor will seek the help of a cardiac specialist, who might then consider a number of tests and introduce an angiotensin-converting enzyme in very low dosages under observation in hospital.

As you can see, all levels of blood-pressure can be controlled since there is a comprehensive and very effective battery of drugs to help you.

A word of warning, however. *Never* take any of these drugs without the fullest consultation with your doctor. If properly used they can prolong life, but indiscriminate and careless drug-taking can have quite the opposite effect. Report any worrying or unwanted side-effects immediately to your doctor.

Chapter 6

Cardiac Research and Technology

Doctors should perhaps not venture into the business of prediction, but on this occasion I will indulge myself. My prophecy is two-fold. First, while medical science will not 'beat' heart disease by providing a cure or a treatment for all forms of cardiac malfunction, it will relegate it from its position as number-one killer in the Western World to a far more lowly position in the lethal league table. Secondly, research into heart disease – by which I mean both fundamental research into the basic causes of heart conditions as well as applied investigations into treatments

and preventive measures – will continue its dramatically accelerating momentum. In the eyes of the general public, the Holy Grail of medicine may well be a comprehensive antidote to cancer, but long before this is attained heart researchers will have achieved many of their most sought-after goals.

Why am I so optimistic? After all, you may well say, coronary heart disease relentlessly continues to scythe down men and women in the prime of life – whatever advice the medical soothsayers throw at us. It is all very well talking about 'changing habits' and 'improved diagnosis' or 'more powerful drugs', but the spectre of heart disease still looms, ready to pounce without warning. But I am sure that we are on the way to beating our public enemy number one. I have not only spent many years of my life treating my own patients and pursuing my own research, but have also looked around at what others are doing. As I take stock of all this zealous effort, I am infected by the overall enthusiasm. Not that I am offering jam today or even tomorrow. But soon…

Genetic research

First let us consider the advances being made in our understanding of what actually *causes* heart disease, both inherited and acquired. As discussed earlier in this book, susceptibility to certain diseases, including CHD, is, to a greater or lesser degree, determined by genetic factors. Anomalies in the microscopic collection of genes within the nucleus of the living cell can be reflected in illnesses that affect the whole person. In the past few years – and all this is very recent indeed – scientists have made enormous strides in understanding the action and purpose of genes, to the extent of being able, in some cases, to manipulate them by using recombinant-DNA technology; the field as a whole is known as 'genetic engineering'.

Two aspects of coronary disease in particular have been subjected to attention by the medical geneticists: the turnover of fatty substances in the blood – lipid metabolism – and the natural factors that influence blood clotting. Researchers are engaged in trying to identify the specific genes that control these processes with a view to making copies of them by the process of cloning. When this has been achieved, they will then have 'gene probes' by which to assess the importance of individual genes in CHD – and to see how it runs in families. Ultimately these delicate, state-of-the-art techniques will be used to build up a genetic 'risk profile' for CHD and thus to establish which individuals are in the greatest danger.

Imagine the advantages of being able to identify an at-risk person long before any symptoms of heart disease begin to show themselves. A doctor would then be able to give

DNA – the key to life.

advice on diet or drug therapies appropriate to minimize a genetically determined pre-disposition to heart disease. We would be closing the stable door long before the horse had even thought of bolting!

Advances in immunology

Another research area that seems to me to be increasingly fruitful is immunology: the study of our natural bodily defence mechanisms. Combined with genetics and virology (the study of virus infections) immunological advances will be of enormous benefit in understanding heart disease. It is predicted that, by using a genetic manipulation technique for producing so-called monoclonal antibodies (highly specific cells that react with particular proteins), researchers will be able to unravel how certain forms of heart disease originate – particularly those associated

An electron micrograph of a cell nucleus. The dark discs on either side of the nucleus are lipids.

with rheumatic fever, myocarditis and inflammatory disorders.

Further advances in immunology will also, I feel, finally enable us to conquer the bane of transplant surgery, rejection. By understanding precisely how and why the body finds a transplanted organ hostile or 'antigenic', it will become possible to suppress these precise responses by drug therapies. Also, I see immunology as one of the routes to preventing and treating severe inflammation occurring in

The production of monoclonal antibodies.

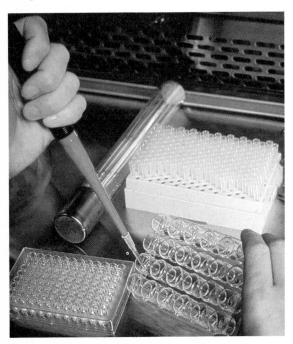

chronic cardiovascular diseases, and new generations of drugs are on the horizon to curb inflammation caused by immune responses.

Virus: a precipitator?

Are some heart attacks caused by a virus infection? This idea has been around for some time, but it is only recently that precise evidence has been offered in support of the viral hypothesis. Dr. Joseph Melnick, at the Baylor College of Medicine in Texas, took samples of diseased arterial tissue from patients undergoing surgery to relieve the blockages caused by thromboses. He found that 25 percent of all his samples showed evidence of infection by a cytomegalovirus – CMV – a very common virus. The CMV organism has, it seems, a capacity for hiding itself within the body – possibly in the arterial walls – where it stays dormant, not actively reproducing. It is not entirely clear how the mechanism that causes blockages works, but the association has been undeniably established.

Further work in this direction could well produce some important clinical payoffs: the prevention of some arterial diseases, perhaps, by immunization; and a more complete understanding of how smoking and cholesterol work alongside an intrusive virus to play their part in the disease process.

New diagnostic approaches

Heart attacks often seem to strike from out of nowhere. Even if you thought you were a candidate for one, you might go along to your doctor or cardiologist only to find that your

Electron micrograph of a pair of cytomegaloviruses.

Digital diagnosis. A computer image of the left ventricle showing nuclear count rate.

ECG reading gave no indication of what was in store. The reason may be that, in the calm conditions of the hospital or doctor's room, your ECG reading is being taken while you are relaxed, lying down and generally unstressed, whereas in reality it is precisely the frenzied, stressful hurly-burly of everyday life that may trigger off an infarct. To get around this, in 1961 a US scientist named Norman Holter introduced the idea of ambulatory monitoring, using a machine that collected a heart record continuously for 24 hours, or longer if required. Holter's first machines weighed a heart-wrenching 22·5kg, but nowadays ambulatory monitors such as the newly launched 'Surveyor' are microminiaturized. In the future I expect to see many more of these machines in clinical services. They are getting faster, cheaper and more cost-effective all the time. Today it is possible to review a whole 24 hours of heart activity in as little as four minutes – a very short time indeed in which to scan for rhythm disturbances and other abnormalities.

Another fascinating piece of hardware is one recently announced by the American Heart Association and being tested by Dr. Gene Bond, pathologist at the Gray School of Medicine in Winston-Salem, North Carolina. An ultrasound detector locates the build-up of fatty deposits in the arteries, carrying out this task without breaking the skin. Here, for the first time, is a non-invasive technique to detect the plaque that causes atherosclerosis before it has built up to thick, hard, clogging proportions.

So far the ultrasound detector has been used only on the carotid arteries in the neck to monitor for signs of stroke; it cannot yet be used to detect coronary atherosclerosis because the relevant area is obscured by the overlying breastbone. But ultrasound clearly has a big future in cardiology. For instance, 'Doppler ultrasound' can be used to measure the speed and turbulence of blood flowing through arteries, so that congested areas can be pinpointed and the relevant information immediately displayed on a computer screen. As new and better machines are developed, it may become possible to scan for all kinds of cardiovascular disorders simply by passing a probe over the outside of the body. 'A non-invasive autopsy' is still for all practical purposes in the realms of cardiological science fiction, but it may not remain there for long.

Still somewhat in its infancy but soon likely to come of age is another non-invasive technique for use in the diagnosis of cardiovascular disorders, nuclear magnetic resonance – NMR. This works by picking up the minute signals produced by the atoms of living tissue as they align themselves under the influence of a strong magnetic field. NMR thus gives the doctor a three-dimensional picture of internal structures without any necessity for the body to be cut open. It is likely to be the future method for mass screening of whole populations for coronary artery disease.

ADVANCES IN DRUG THERAPY AND SELF HEALING

Because digitalis (see Chapter 4) can be poisonous if given in amounts only slightly greater than those needed to be therapeutic, researchers have been exploring the possibility of alternatives, such as Milrinone. This drug is currently being evaluated experimentally (which means it is some way off being used with patients on a widespread basis) at the Beth Israel Hospital in Boston by Dr. Donald Bain. Writing in the *New England Journal of Medicine* about his research, in which he tried Milrinone on 80 patients with congestive heart disease, Dr. Bain concluded: 'If its lack of side-effects are borne out in larger-scale trials then... Milrinone will revolutionize the treatment of heart failure.' The drug functions partly by dilating the arteries but may also have direct effects on the heart itself. It is a highly promising development.

In addition to advances with new drugs, researchers are studying self-healing mechanisms. The heart has an amazing capacity to recover and heal itself after a heart attack. Dead muscle is quickly replaced by scar tissue and new capillaries slowly grow into these areas – a process called angiogeneisis.

Researchers have reasoned that, if angiogeneisis could be understood, they might be able to encourage recovery by natural means. They have identified a substance – the 'angiogeneisis factor' – that seems to be implicated in the process. Apparently the heart itself produces this chemical when needed for its own recovery.

The next step is to find out more about the angiogeneisis factor: how it works, what it is made of, and whether it might be the basis of a new drug to speed recovery.

Prostaglandins

Also promising is research on prostaglandins, a group of substances, first identified nearly 50 years ago, which occur naturally in the body. Current research into prostaglandins – which is still at an early stage – reveals that these biologically active compounds have effects on both the behaviour of blood platelets and the calibre of blood vessels – two factors that are, of course, critical in the formation of thromboses.

One type of prostaglandin – thromboxane – seems to cause platelet-aggregation and vasoconstriction, while another – prostacyclin – seems to have quite opposite effects, inhibiting platelet-aggregation and causing vasodilation.

(a) Clumps of platelets (left) reacting with the vessel wall without prostacyclin; (b) shows how prostacyclin prevents platelets from clumping together.

As both these actions might be manipulated to therapeutic effect, researchers have, as you might expect, been trying to find ways to increase the natural production of prostacyclin and decrease that of thromboxane. The task so far has been far from easy, even discouraging, but I am reassured by these words from Dr. A. M. Breckenridge, Professor of Pharmacology at Liverpool University: 'So far this has proved frustratingly difficult, but new pharmacological tools (either novel agents or old drugs such as aspirin given in low doses) hold promise.' (Breckenridge, A.,M., 'Five years back and five years forward', in *Cardiovascular Research*, 1983, British Heart Foundation.)

One type of prostaglandin – the so-called 'E-type' – has also proved invaluable in pediatric cardiology. Its use is becoming practically routine treatment for newborn babies with congenital heart disease whose pulmonary or systemic circulation is dependent on the action of the ductus arteriosus. E-type can rapidly reduce cyanosis in newborns with ductus-dependent circulation by preventing spontaneous closure of the duct.

Calcium blockers

Another fruitful research area in drug treatments concerns the so-called calcium-channel-blocking agents, or calcium blockers. Calcium is an important natural factor in all types of muscle contraction – and that includes in the walls of blood vessels and in the myocardium. Now certain drugs can stop calcium entering the cells of the walls of coronary vessels, and these have been shown to be valuable treatments for a whole range of heart disorders: ischemic heart disease, arrhythmias, hypertension and heart failure.

There are many subgroups of calcium blockers, some of which are more specific for

a

b

(a) A filter taken from a heart-lung machine during a cardiopulmonary bypass operation showing platelet aggregation partially occluding the filter pores, and (b) a filter taken from a similar operation where prostacyclin has been added to the circulation, clearly showing how prostacyclin prevents platelet aggregation.

heart-rhythm control, others for preventing spasm and enabling the blood vessels to relax (vasodilation), thus reducing blood pressure. So far much of this work has been confined to the laboratory benches of the experimenters, but I expect it to flower eventually in the form of whole new generations of useful drugs. At the moment we can only guess at the potential of the calcium blockers.

HI-TECH TREATMENTS

By combining sound medical skills with advances in electronics, physics, biochemistry and a whole host of other specialities – both biological and technological – the heart specialists of today have made some almost incredible leaps forward in the treatment of various types of heart disease. Even as you read this, someone, somewhere is no doubt inching the whole enterprise a little further on, pushing to the limits the feasible and the practical.

Balloon angioplasty

This technique does not require open-heart surgery, and so is rapidly gaining popularity. A catheter with a tiny balloon in its tip is slipped through a peripheral artery into the area of a constriction in the coronary artery. Once there, the balloon is inflated, thereby pushing out the narrowed walls and crushing the fatty plaque tissue. The progress of the catheter is watched all the way on a television screen. At present this method is used only for limited and fairly localized disease.

The procedure takes perhaps an hour and is performed under local anaesthesia and sedation, so the patient may return home after only three days in hospital and commence work virtually immediately. This treatment is particularly suited to patients who have a critical narrowing in only one artery – a stenosis threatening a heart attack. It is also valuable for those patients who could not tolerate a full coronary-bypass graft operation, perhaps because they are elderly or have associated lung disease which raises the risk of formal surgery. This balloon technique

A nuclear-powered artificial heart.

has been used also to clear blocked valves in the heart – balloon valvuloplasty.

Laser artery cleaning

This is an experimental procedure, at the moment mainly confined to laboratory animals but with considerable potential for human patients. The idea is to guide a laser beam along a blocked artery to burn away fatty deposits.

A variation of this type of microsurgery is to guide a laser beam along optical fibres to the wall of the ventricles, where it can drill tiny holes and thereby allow blood to flow from the cavity to the heart muscle. This form of revascularization is being tested at the moment, and, if it works, it will be useful for some, though not all, patients with ischemic heart disease. As an operation it has one enormous merit: it takes only five minutes as compared to the hours required to do conventional bypass.

To date, laser angioplasty has been tried on very few patients and is thus still highly experimental. Drugs such as streptokinase, squirted along a catheter, are more often used for these exercises in arterial vacuum-cleaning. However, laser techniques are fast developing and I expect to see them in more widespread use before long.

Balloon pumps

These are not really 'experimental' as such; they are increasingly used in the USA, where an estimated 30 000 are temporarily inserted each year. Again, I expect to see this treatment more extensively employed. The balloon pump, invented by Dr. Adrian Kantrowitz in the mid-1960s provides aid to a weakened – indeed dying – heart. It consists of a catheter which is inserted into an artery in the groin and fed up to the aorta. At the end is a fine, 25 cm-long sausage-shaped balloon. Helium is pumped into the balloon and out again with a pulsing rhythm, causing it to expand and collapse. This augments the pumping action of the heart, reducing the workload on the muscle and improving coronary blood flow. Thus a patient can be kept alive with a pump for months if necessary, until, say, bypass surgery can be performed to unblock the clogged arteries on a more-or-less permanent basis.

Incidentally, these balloon pumps have also been of importance in showing how an implanted machine can keep the body going for a time. This is paving the way for experiments on artificial hearts, such as the device that was given to Barney Clark (see Chapter 4).

Dr. Adrian Kantrowitz and his team at the Sinai Hospital in Detroit have been working on the sorts of problems that beset artificial-heart implantation, especially the tendency to infection. If a balloon pump is left in place for a long

Dr. W. De Vries (arms folded) ready to implant an artificial heart.

time, it is possible that infectious bacteria may enter the flesh along the tube that carries the helium. Dr. Kantrowitz is working on a kind of plastic skin-plug that will provide a congenial home for natural skin-cells, so that the skin-cells will grow into the plastic and create a germ-tight seal. Animal experiments to date have been promising, and I look forward to further results – this time with human patients.

And the future...

Other technological developments on the horizon include the refinement of pacemakers to the extent that the patient will be wearing both a monitoring device and a heart-rhythm sustainer, the two instruments being combined and computer-controlled. The patient will wear an implantable device which will monitor and analyse abnormal rhythms and send these data to a cardiac centre; the device will also be controllable from the local hospital by radio, so that doctors there can carry out the appropriate therapy without even seeing the patient. Thus the heart's pace can be monitored, checked, regulated and improved by one system. Automatically and without fuss.

Part II

Keeping Healthy

Introduction

Despite all the continuing advances made in the healing of sick hearts, we must acknowledge the importance of preventing heart disease in the first place. There are five simple routes to keeping your heart healthy: coping with stress, care over diet and weight, regular exercise, abstinence from smoking, and caution over alcohol. It is all very well to patch up a battered heart or even swap it for a new one, but acquired heart disease is now regarded as one of the most avoidable ailments in the Western World, and because so many contributing factors are connected to habit and lifestyle, every effort should be made to provide sensible, non-alarmist information about prevention, not only for adults but for young people as well.

Children need to be made aware of how their bodies work, and of the various ways of adjusting to and adopting a healthy way of life. It is common sense that we should learn this while still young, in the home and in the school. Much attention has recently been drawn to evidence showing that a build-up of fatty deposits in the arteries can occur long before adulthood; if children have, say, unbalanced diets, or start smoking at school, a lifetime of bad habits can ensue – thus increasing the risk of heart trouble and other problems. Educating children's bodies beyond the simple rigours of school sports and physical education is vital if the high toll in heart victims is to be reduced.

As well as providing a health programme at school level, improvements in nutrition are necessary. Beefburgers and other high-fat junk foods are increasingly present on school menus, but parents can play a large part in prevention by giving their children more fresh foods at the expense of endless rounds of fried, sugary and processed stodge.

Part II of *Your Healthy Heart* gives a practical guide to staying healthy and living longer – and remember: it's never too early, or too late, to start looking after yourself.

Chapter 7
Controlling Stress

Turn back the clock 30 thousand years and picture the scene that must often have confronted our prehistoric ancestors in their constant search for food and shelter. Entering a forest clearing, the hunter suddenly comes upon a ferocious-looking tiger, prowling around in the hope of catching today's meal. They both stand stock-still, their eyes meet, and within his tensed body the man feels a rapid pounding of the heart, as his mouth goes dry and sweat rolls down his anxious brow. Breathing hard and thinking fast, he has to make a decision: stand and face the possibility of a fight to the death; or turn tail and disappear into the thickets.

This describes a classic example of the mechanism for survival built into us and other animals by millions of years of evolution: fight or flight. And triggering it all off is *stress*.

There is nothing new about stress, nor is it an 'unnatural' phenomenon. Indeed, it is unavoidable in all our lives, just as it was for our prehistoric forerunners. What is new, though, is the level of stress we subject ourselves to: a stone-age system is being constantly buffeted by space-age lifestyles. The biological mechanism is too often forced to cope with the highly geared demands of modern living, many of which are self-inflicted. Although stress is part and parcel of our lives, we are always abusing our capacity to meet its challenges. As a result, while we are not being leapt on by marauding tigers, we are being attacked by rather more insidiously dangerous forces which build up over many years, and culminate in a final assault on that most precious part of us: the heart.

WHAT IS STRESS?

In 1900 the polar explorer Sir Ernest Shackleton put the following advertisement in *The Times* stating: 'Men wanted for hazardous journey. Small wages, bitter cold, long months of complete darkness, constant danger, safe return doubtful. Honour and recognition in case of success.' Not, you might think, an invitation calculated to attract much support! In the event, hundreds of people rushed to reply, demonstrating that what to most of us would be intolerably 'stressful' circumstances were, to them, highly desirable. How would, say, a racing-car driver react to a job behind the counter in a bank? The

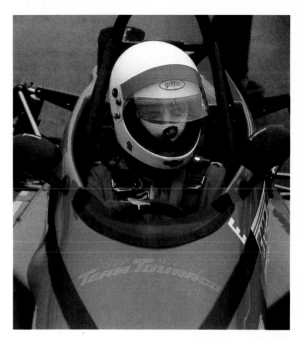
One man's stress is another's excitement.

A typical urban traffic jam. Modern living tends to produce perpetual stress, so that adrenalin is constantly being released.

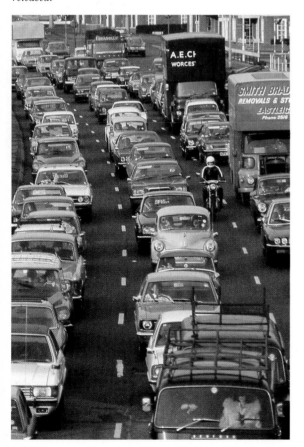

'stress' of all that civilized calm, by contrast with the screaming, smelly excitement and danger of the track, would be intolerable. In other words, stress can be defined not just in terms of excessive demands, but in terms of inappropriate pressures. It can arise when people do things they are not equipped for.

Stress is, therefore, too much of the wrong sort of pressure. It can also be thought of as a reaction to change of any kind. A change is as good as a rest, but if you are not equipped to meet it then the saying is simply incorrect. And

Sports events may get spectators worked up, but also provide release from daily tension.

This scene may be peaceful enough, but it can sometimes be difficult adapting to major changes like retirement – or even taking a vacation.

when I say that change can be stressful, I am not just referring to large-scale, distressing upheavals such as bereavement or divorce. Even pleasant events, such as moving to a better house, may have subtly adverse effects on both mental and physical health.

STRESS AND THE HEART

What are the short-term effects of stress on our heart and circulatory system? As the brain receives a 'stress message', the relevant nerve cells immediately act to stimulate the pituitary gland. This organ then activates other glands to secrete hormones, especially adrenalin, which is the substance that excites various bodily systems, including the heart. Immediately there are increases in systolic blood-pressure, heart-rate and pulse-pressure – along with a whole host of other physiological responses. The heart is working overtime to get blood around the body to those tensed muscles; and the faster it pumps the greater the pressure exerted on the arteries. If the stress subsides, these responses die away. The body can be released from the tensions to return to a state of equilibrium. Thus athletes build themselves up to a state of induced stress for an important event, and afterwards their bodies subside back to the resting state.

What happens to someone who is constantly in a condition of high stress? Instead of returning to that desirable post-stress phase, the body *adapts* to the pressures so that the fight-or-flight changes in physiological response become a permanent feature. High blood-pressure, constricted blood vessels, a pounding heart and exceptional circulation start to take over. Under these circumstances we begin to harm the heart and its attendant systems. Also, we begin to run even harder to 'keep up', because we are fighting growing feelings of inadequacy and anxiety, which are themselves stressful, and increase the level of bodily excitation.

Ultimately we reach a critical point which a leading British cardiologist, Dr. Peter Nixon, has identified as the 'exhaustion curve'. Instead of improving our performance under stress, we reach a point where greater pressure is actually counterproductive and produces breakdown. We have slipped down a vicious exhaustion spiral. This is the sort of situation which could give rise to a stress-induced heart attack.

The causes and the evidence
There is some debate among scientists as to how this may happen. Do we succumb because stress

Electrodes fitted for stress testing.

People with too much work and monotony and too little reward or recognition often become victims of stress-related heart problems.

A dangerous job induces a different kind of stress to repetitive, 'safer' work.

One of the most stressful occupations of all: housewife and mother.

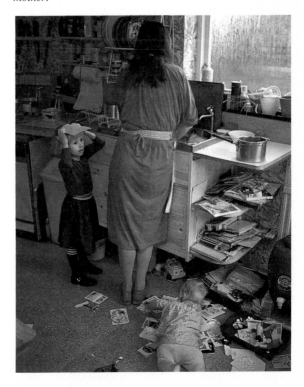

has kept our blood-pressure up over a long period? Or can stress have an even more direct effect? Researchers at the Atherosclerosis Research Center in the USA carried out some experiments with laboratory monkeys to find out how stress-induced heart attacks are caused. They took two groups of animals and fed them both on a low-fat, low-cholesterol diet and matched them for body-weight and blood-pressure readings. They then subjected one group to high levels of stress, in this case by making them live in cages that broke up their normal social groupings, while the others were allowed to fraternize naturally. At the end of the experiment, 21 months after starting, the stressed monkeys were found to have serious signs of fatty deposits in their arteries. This happened despite the fact that the monkeys were kept on a healthy diet and at a healthy weight. In other words, there was positive evidence of heart disease induced by stress – quite independently of other lifestyle factors. If this much is true in experimental monkeys, who are close relatives to mankind in the family of animals, could the same be true for us? I am inclined to agree with the experimenters' view that, though not conclusive, their findings are highly suggestive. Interestingly enough, the *Lancet* carried an article in 1983 reporting that the incidence of fatal heart attacks rose sharply in the city of Athens in the days after the 1981 earthquake. The heart-stress connection seems too powerful to ignore.

The social-readjustment rating scale

LIFE EVENT	SCORE	
1 Death of spouse	100	☐
2 Divorce	73	☐
3 Marital separation from mate	65	☐
4 Detention in jail or other institution	63	☐
5 Death of a close family member	63	☐
6 Major personal injury or illness	53	☐
7 Marriage	50	☐
8 Being fired from work	47	☐
9 Marital reconciliation with mate	45	☐
10 Retirement from work	45	☐
11 Major change in the health or behaviour of a family member	44	☐
12 Pregnancy	40	☐
13 Sexual difficulties	39	☐
14 Gaining a new family member (e.g., through birth, adoption, oldster moving in)	39	☐
15 Major business readjustment (e.g., merger, reorganization, bankruptcy)	39	☐
16 Major change in financial state (e.g., a lot worse off or a lot better off than usual)	38	☐
17 Death of a close friend	37	☐
18 Changing to a different line of work	36	☐
19 Major change in the number of arguments with spouse (either a lot more or a lot less than usual regarding child-rearing, personal habits, etc.)	35	☐
20 Taking on a mortgage (or purchasing a home, business, etc.)	31	☐
21 Foreclose on a mortgage or loan	30	☐
22 Major change in responsibilities at work (e.g., promotion, demotion, lateral transfer)	29	☐
23 Son/daughter leaving home (e.g., marriage, attending college)	29	☐

ARE YOU UNDER STRESS?

We know the dangers are out there, but what can we do about them? My anti-stress campaign really falls into two phases: first we have to try to identify the stresses in our lives and assess whether they are potentially harmful; secondly, we have to tailor a plan for coping with those

stresses that do fall into the dangerous or even lethal category.

Two doctors, T. Holmes and R. Rahe, working at the Naval Neuropsychiatric Unit in San Diego, California, began to ponder on the kinds of experiences that might be stressful, and indeed whether there was a kind of 'league table' of life events that they could draw up for future

LIFE EVENT		SCORE	
24	In-law troubles	29	☐
25	Outstanding personal achievement	28	☐
26	Wife beginning or ceasing work outside the home	26	☐
27	Beginning or ceasing formal schooling	26	☐
28	Major change in living conditions (e.g., building a new home, remodelling, deterioration of home or neighbourhood)	25	☐
29	Revision of personal habits (dress, manners, associations, etc.)	24	☐
30	Troubles with the boss	24	☐
31	Major change in working hours or conditions	20	☐
32	Change in residence	20	☐
33	Change to a new school	20	☐
34	Major change in usual type and/or amount of recreation	19	☐
35	Major change in church activities (e.g., a lot more or less than usual)	19	☐
36	Major change in social activities (e.g., clubs, dancing, movies, visiting)	18	☐
37	Taking on a mortgage or loan (e.g., for purchasing a car, TV, freezer)	17	☐
38	Major change in sleeping habits (a lot more or a lot less sleep, or a change in the time of day when asleep)	16	☐
39	Major change in number of family get-togethers (e.g., a lot more or a lot less than usual)	15	☐
40	Major change in eating habits (a lot more or a lot less food intake, or very different hours for or surroundings during meals)	15	☐
41	Vacation	15	☐
42	Christmas	12	☐
43	Minor violations of the law (e.g., traffic tickets, jaywalking, disturbing the peace)	11	☐

Source: T. Holmes and R. Rahe, 'The Social Readjustment Scale', in Journal of Psychosomatic Research, vol. 11, 1967

guidance. What emerged was the celebrated Holmes-Rahe social-readjustment rating scale. Rahe found that myocardial infarction was frequently preceded by an abrupt change of circumstance three to six months before the attack. He also noted that, the greater the change, the shorter the time that elapsed before the onset of the attack, and the more likely was the risk of sudden death from the infarct.

To find out whether you are possibly at risk, all you have to do is check off on the scale each of the life events that has happened to you over the past year, then add up the total number of points as indicated in the right-hand column.

Holmes and Rahe found that people with a tally of 300 or over in any one year had an 80 percent

Job stress check	No stress at all					A great deal of stress
My relationship with my boss	0	1	2	3	4	5
My relationships with my colleagues	0	1	2	3	4	5
My relationships with my subordinates	0	1	2	3	4	5
Workload	0	1	2	3	4	5
Making mistakes	0	1	2	3	4	5
Feeling undervalued	0	1	2	3	4	5
Time pressures and deadlines	0	1	2	3	4	5
Promotion prospects	0	1	2	3	4	5
Rate of pay	0	1	2	3	4	5
Demands of work on my private life	0	1	2	3	4	5
My spouse's attitude towards my work	0	1	2	3	4	5
The amount of travel required by my work	0	1	2	3	4	5

chance of succumbing to some form of medical condition (not just heart problems) within about two years. For those whose score was in the 150–300 range, the chances were about evens. People below this level – who qualified as having had 'low' life-change scores – had a 30 percent chance of illness.

But do not think that, if you have a high score, you will automatically succumb to some mortal disease. After all, events such as divorce and marriage are pretty commonplace, and no one is suggesting that walking up to the altar or out of the lawyer's office is tantamount to taking the quick road to a coronary. There are many other factors to take into account.

JOB STRESS AND THE HEART

First a conundrum. Why is it that US presidents tend to live longer than vice-presidents? Why

	No stress at all					A great deal of stress
Being relocated	0	1	2	3	4	5
Taking work home	0	1	2	3	4	5
Managing people	0	1	2	3	4	5
Office politics	0	1	2	3	4	5
Lack of power and influence	0	1	2	3	4	5
My beliefs conflicting with those of the company	0	1	2	3	4	5
Lack of consultation and communication in my company	0	1	2	3	4	5
Clarity of my job	0	1	2	3	4	5
Conflict between my work group and others in the organization	0	1	2	3	4	5
Top management does not understand my work-related problems	0	1	2	3	4	5

Source: C.L. Cooper, The Stress Check, Prentice-Hall, 1981

should the most influential man in the most powerful country in the world, whose finger controls the nuclear button, fare better than his deputy, cushioned from a mass of seemingly insoluble problems by being an understudy? The answer probably lies right there. The vice-president is an also-ran, a passenger, an observer, while the president is in the driving seat: he has succeeded. Success may promote longevity, giving you something real to live for.

Coronary heart disease, some people would say, is far more likely to hit the middle-manager, the person thrusting but still not quite reaching the executive summits, than those lofty souls who inhabit boardrooms and take all the very big decisions. Another stress-related heart sufferer is the ambitious person who has no perspective on their own limitations, believing they can do it all. If they fail to achieve their desired goals, they refuse to settle for second best.

Checking stress

Now let's get down to the nitty-gritty of deciding whether your job is more than just taxing, energy-consuming or whatever. Let's see whether it really does qualify for the description 'stressful'. In the job stress questionnaire you have to circle the number that best describes the

amount of stress you experience in various situations represented by the statements in the left-hand column. Be as fair as you can – and be honest with yourself!

If you score 4 or 5 on any of the items you may wish to think about taking some action. A substantial proportion of high scores means that

Stressful work conditions

		Never	Rarely	Sometimes	Often	Always
1	Others I work with seem unclear about what my job is	1	2	3	4	5
2	I have differences of opinion with my superiors	1	2	3	4	5
3	Others' demands for my time at work are in conflict with each other	1	2	3	4	5
4	I lack confidence in 'management'	1	2	3	4	5
5	'Management' expects me to interrupt my work for new priorities	1	2	3	4	5
6	There is conflict between my unit and others it must work with	1	2	3	4	5
7	I only get feedback when my performance is unsatisfactory	1	2	3	4	5
8	Decisions or changes which affect me are made 'above' without my knowledge or involvement	1	2	3	4	5
9	I have too much to do and too little time to do it	1	2	3	4	5
10	I feel over qualified for the work I actually do	1	2	3	4	5
11	I feel under qualified for the work I actually do	1	2	3	4	5
12	The people I work closely with are trained in a different field than mine	1	2	3	4	5
13	I must go to other departments to get my job done	1	2	3	4	5
14	I have unsettled conflicts with people in my department	1	2	3	4	5
15	I have unsettled conflicts with other departments	1	2	3	4	5
16	I get little personal support from the people I work with	1	2	3	4	5
17	I spend my time 'fighting fires' rather than working to a plan	1	2	3	4	5
18	Management misunderstands the real needs of my department in the organization	1	2	3	4	5
19	I feel family pressure about long hours, weekend work, etc	1	2	3	4	5

remedial action is essential.

Having completed the job stress check you should now move on to the actual conditions under which you are currently working, and fill in the related stressful work conditions questionnaire below. Circle the number to describe the degree of stress you think you are experiencing, working down the items one by one. Again the watchword is honesty. The whole object of the exercise is to get you to evaluate your own problems. There are no passes or fails in this test. If you have a significant number of high scores, my anti-stress programme should be beneficial.

		Never	Rarely	Sometimes	Often	Always
20	Self-imposed demand to meet scheduled deadlines	1	2	3	4	5
21	I have difficulty giving negative feedback to peers	1	2	3	4	5
22	I have difficulty giving negative feedback to subordinates	1	2	3	4	5
23	I have difficulty in dealing with aggressive people	1	2	3	4	5
24	I have difficulty dealing with passive people	1	2	3	4	5
25	Overlapping responsibilities cause me problems	1	2	3	4	5
26	I am uncomfortable arbitrating a conflict among my peers	1	2	3	4	5
27	I am uncomfortable arbitrating a conflict among my subordinates	1	2	3	4	5
28	Academic and administrative roles are in conflict	1	2	3	4	5
29	I avoid conflicts with peers	1	2	3	4	5
30	I avoid conflicts with superiors	1	2	3	4	5
31	I avoid conflicts with subordinates	1	2	3	4	5
32	Allocation of resources generates conflict in my organization	1	2	3	4	5
33	I experience frustration with conflicting procedures	1	2	3	4	5
34	My personal needs are in conflict with the organization	1	2	3	4	5
35	My professional expertise contradicts organizational practice	1	2	3	4	5
36	Administrative policies inhibit getting the job done	1	2	3	4	5
37	Other	1	2	3	4	5

Source: J. Steinmetz, 'The stress-reduction program at University Hospital, University of California Medical Center, San Diego', Proceedings of the Conference on Occupational Stress, sponsored by the National Institute of Occupational Safety and Health, November 1977

THE ANTI-STRESS PROGRAMME

By now, I hope, you will have a better understanding of those factors in your personal and working life that are potentially stressful, and the physical and mental symptoms that could mean that something is amiss. Having recognized the enemy, it is your turn to fight back with my Three-point Anti-stress Programme.

One: know your own personality

In his fascinating studies of the behaviour under stress of individuals in wartime or subjected to brainwashing procedures, the celebrated UK psychiatrist William Sargant recognized that people varied in their ability to cope with various stressful situations according to their temperament. He found that men of 'phlegmatic temperament', who were well adjusted and had a settled, happy outlook on life, were likely to hold out longer than those who did not possess these assets. In other words, it is important to know

Type A people are more aggressive, ambitious and angry – and may be hurrying on the road to a heart attack.

what sort of a person you are in order to discover the degree of stress or the type of stress you can withstand. The world's leading stress expert, Hans Selye, puts it thus:

> The goal is certainly not to avoid stress… there is no more justification for avoiding stress than for shunning food, exercise or love. But in order to express yourself fully you must first find your optimum stress level.

How are we to do this? In my view the best guidelines come from Dr. Ray Rosemann and Dr. Meyer Friedman, two cardiologists who, several decades ago, showed that coronary-prone people were what they called 'Type A' personalities – driving, competitive, obsessive, aggressive characters who are typical workaholics, always in a hurry in the office, at home or in a restaurant. In contrast to the clock-watching 'Type A' is the 'Type B', easy-going, placid, relaxed, ready to take time off to do very little, and not really interested in keeping up with the Joneses or anyone else.

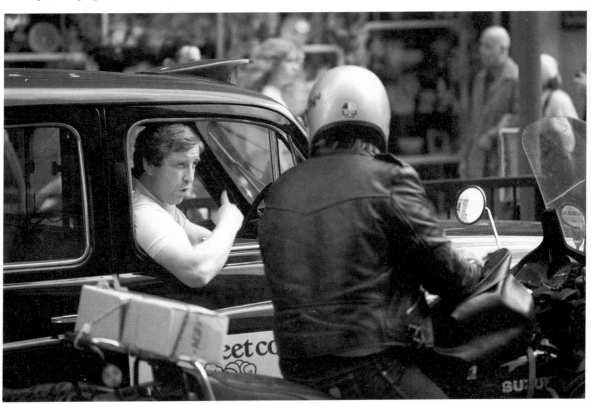

Are you a Type A?

How well do you recognize yourself from this profile? Are you:

Easily irritated? ☐

Guilty about relaxing? ☐

Impatient with people? ☐

Taking on excessive responsibilities? ☐

Attempting to master the unmasterable? ☐

Upset when things turn out badly? ☐

A loner? ☐

Bad at resolving family problems? ☐

Always pressed for time? ☐

Working on a hundred things at once? ☐

A workaholic? ☐

Bad at relaxing during leisure-time such as holidays? ☐

A quick eater, rapid talker, jerky mover? ☐

If you have one or more of these traits, then just think about the relationship that has been established between Type A behaviour and heart disease. Look at the Table, which outlines characteristics of Type As and their relative susceptibilities to coronary problems, drawn up after a large-scale study in California over the course of 10 years.

If you are a Type A personality it is, of course, very difficult to change your innate characteristics. But you can at least recognize that you are one of those in the danger zone of stress-related illness and be firm with yourself about making adjustments to your life to lessen your personal susceptibilities. In fact the more 'yes' answers you gave to the questions about Type A personality, the more pronounced those adjustments will have to be, and the more urgently you will have to make them. This brings me to the second arm of my anti-stress campaign.

Two: choose an appropriate response to stress

Because stress is essentially a *reaction*, and because we all react differently to different situations, you have to tailor any attempts to combat stress to meet your personal requirements and circumstances. For specific guidelines you should consult the section on relaxation later in this chapter, but there are certain general points that anyone and everyone should follow:

Avoid getting overtired by keeping a nice balance between rest and activity.

Make sure that you give yourself the time, conditions and frame of mind to ensure enough good-quality sleep.

Cultivate the ability to say 'no' to demands put on you if you feel that these are going to cause you to feel overburdened.

Don't be afraid to admit your limitations: we all have them, but only you can decide in all honesty where your own limits lie.

Keep a 'stress diary', in which you note your particularly stressful times during the week: by spotting the critical periods you will be able to apply anti-tension, relaxation measures when they are needed to reduce your unwanted responses.

Never be shy about seeking help and advice about stressful situations: one of the problems with stress is that it can be self-reinforcing.

If you worry unduly about a chest pain, imagining that it indicates 'a bad heart', make a quick visit to the doctor: you will probably find that there is nothing to worry about.

A CHD relaxation programme – the Californian connection shows the benefits

Researchers at the Recurrent Coronary Prevention Program in California set these goals for lifestyle changes in coronary patients. Achieving some of them over a three-year period has halved the rate of second heart attacks among 600 sufferers.

BEHAVIOURAL: **what I do**

Speech: talk slower, interrupt less, less emphasis in talking.
Listening: reflect and paraphrase more. Focus full attention on other person(s).
Psychomotor: less abrupt gesturing with head and hands. Less fidgeting and jiggling. Smile and laugh more: look for the humour in things.
Waiting: practise waiting with more patience (e.g., in bank, restaurant, post office, supermarket, department store, traffic jam); use waiting time to reflect.
Modelling: practise acting in a more Type B manner for others to see.

ENVIRONMENTAL: **where I live and with whom**

Spend time physically relaxing – 20 minutes a day. Have a regular 'discuss/review' time with spouse – at least once a month for 30 minutes.

Reduce TV watching of violent, highly competitive or disturbing events (e.g., football matches, the news).

Do *not* take on new or additional tasks without at least reducing current tasks (no 'add-ons'). Discuss new tasks with group.

Drive more slowly (55 mph/90 kph), and stay in the right lane. Speak more often with neighbours; take time to be friendly.

COGNITIVE: **what and how I think**

Ask myself each day: 'What am I denying?'

Remind myself daily that the way I perceive (see) things (not the things themselves) is the problem to be solved.

Use my feelings (e.g., anger) to examine my beliefs about what has happened (e.g., someone criticized me).

Notice my 'self-talk' and see how it fits certain beliefs or fears; practise positive self-talk.

Practise self-instructions to reduce stress in anticipated (although individually unexpected) situations.

Reduce seeing what happens (events, persons) as direct challenges or threats.

PHYSIOLOGICAL: **how I feel and what my body is doing**

Minimize heavy or large meals with foods high in fats.

Eat more often during the day instead of having one meal at the end of the day.

Comply with prescribed medication.

Carry nitroglycerine.

Avoid running or jogging, unless medically supervised with defibrillator.

Source: Quoted in Wood, C., 'Relax, and stop a heart attack', *New Scientist,* vol. 100, no. 1379, 1983

However, according to Dr. Charles Speilberger of the University of Southern Florida, we can go further than this general division into Types A and B. Speilberger, a leading authority on stress-related diseases, reckons that a vital component of coronary-prone behaviour is what might be called a tendency towards rage reactions. The high-risk people are those who, if they feel they are being unfairly criticized, react with a high degree of anger and hostility. They magnify the adverse reactions of other people through this prism of rage, and their fury seems to double back on them and promote dangerous bodily symptoms. Even if they explode with anger, gaining emotional release, there is no such release for their heart and cardiovascular system. Control over one's own anger is therefore something one should aim for. And this is where relaxation techniques, especially quickie methods such as deep breathing or even a warm shower, come into their own. Of course,

Peaceful surroundings have a calming effect away from the rough and tumble of city life.

the multiplicity of seemingly insoluble problems in a person's life are bound to cause stress. But if you acknowledge its existence, you have taken the first step in coming to terms with it even in the midst of life's difficulties.

Three: your life in your hands

When you come to analyse what it is in life that stresses you, you find that it is often just a question of time-management. You are capable of doing things but not necessarily at the time – and within the time – allocated for them. To perform a tricky heart operation all day in the theatre is demanding, right enough, but would I call it stressful? Probably not – because I am doing something I love, surrounded by a supportive and skilled team, and trying to help another person live a longer and fuller life. That is rewarding. Invigorating. What really stresses me are demands such as the need to attend finance-committee meetings or deal with urgent administrative problems when my mind is on medical matters. Trying to do too many things at once, or having to sacrifice what you want to do for what you need to do – these are the real stress factors.

But, once more, they can be combated. Take, for instance, the busy executive: the bustling time-stressed individual, eating too much and drinking too regularly, always on the upward-thrusting go. Hundreds of his type have been in my cardiac wards. If only they had applied some of their undoubted intelligence and logistic skill to managing their own lives better!

A leading authority on this type of frenzied, self-denying behaviour, Professor Cary Cooper, offers a simple guide (below) for coping with job stress which one might well apply with profit outside the office.

RELAXATION – PRINCIPLES AND PRACTICES

I like to have a dog around the house: dogs show us what true relaxation really is. Watch a dog stretching out for a rest: from a position of poised muscles and sharp senses, it suddenly seems to let everything go into a thoroughly calm, inert state of well-being. Within seconds, you can lift its paw and it will drop with a soporific thump. If only we humans could relax so readily.

Relaxation seems to act as a buffer between our bodies and the stresses that drive us into unhealthy paths. A classic demonstration of this was given by a UK general practitioner, Dr. Chandra Patel, who treated 20 patients suffering from raised blood-pressure by using an unusual technique. Instead of just relying on drugs and dietary measures, Dr. Patel got her patients to carry out two 20-minute sessions of relaxation allied to meditation each day. At the same time she studied the progress of another group of patients who were following a more conventional medical regime.

The results were highly convincing. The relaxation group showed dramatic falls in blood pressure over the course of a year, and needed far fewer drugs to maintain their health than the others. Dr. Patel's is not a lone voice. The same improvements in blood-pressure levels have been achieved by Dr. Herbert Benson of the Harvard Medical School using transcendental meditation.

What attracts me to the whole field of relaxation methods is that it is so varied. There are dozens of techniques to choose from. Some

How to handle job stress

TIME MANAGEMENT

Schedule daily uninterruptible organizing time

Make a list of tasks, in order of priority

Set realistic deadlines

Concentrate on one task at a time

Avoid indecisiveness

Consider each problem in depth

Lunch away from the office

Do not neglect family time

Develop a hobby that demands total concentration

Plan leisurely vacations

LEARN TO DELEGATE

Expect the best from people, and give them the benefit of the doubt

Improve communication skills with subordinates and superiors – listen without interruption

Keep your sense of humour

Give negative and positive feedback

Know what is going on

KEEP YOUR SELF-RESPECT

Form realistic personal goals

Learn to accept limitations in yourself

Learn from mistakes and avoid negative self-talk

Source: Thames Television Limited, *How to Last a Lifetime,* 1981

Relaxation is made easier by having a satisfying pastime.

have a spiritual or meditational flavour; some others are purely pragmatic in character. Some are for loners; others are ideal as a group activity. Some can, if you wish, involve studying and deep understanding; others are quick, simple and learned in a trice.

Below is an outline of some of these techniques to give you an idea of where to start if the field is completely new to you – conversely; if you are dissatisfied with your existing relaxation methods, you may find a technique that has greater appeal. Do not be afraid to be experimental: just try what you fancy and drop it after giving it a reasonable run if you find it unproductive. You will know if it is doing you any good without needing to have your blood-pressure readings as evidence. Whichever method you opt for, do not think you have to master it totally before you are entitled to derive any benefits.

Inner peace

Relaxation is all about using your mind to control your body, but that implies that you can reach a calm state of mind in the first place. Learn a simple 'through exercise' method such as the one below to induce mental relaxation whenever it is needed. It will also, of course, have immediate bodily benefits as well.

1 Select a comfortable sitting or reclining position.

2 Close your eyes and think about a place

where you have been before that represents your ideal spot for physical and mental relaxation. (It should be a quiet environment, perhaps the seashore, the mountains, or even your own back garden. If you can't think of an ideal relaxation place, then create one in your mind.)

3 Now imagine that you are actually in your ideal relaxation place. Imagine that you are seeing all the colours, hearing the sounds, smelling the aromas. Just lie back and enjoy your soothing, rejuvenating environment.

4 Feel the peacefulness, the calmness, and imagine your whole body and mind being renewed and refreshed.

5 After five to ten minutes, slowly open your eyes and stretch. You have the realization that you may instantly return to your relaxation place whenever you desire, and experience a peacefulness and calmness in body and mind.

Source: B.B. Brown, *Stress and the Art of Biofeedback*, Bantam Books, 1977

Physical relaxation

Although it may be easier to become relaxed in the quiet comfort of, say, a favourite armchair, the big advantage of the exercises shown here is that you can do them anywhere – such as when you are waiting in a frustrating traffic jam, or for a plane to touch down after a bumpy ride. These are just some of the occasions when I have deployed these methods to enormous effect. They are gentle, soothing and completely safe, even if you have a history of heart disease.

Relaxation, an everyday technique

1 Sit quietly in a comfortable position.

2 Close your eyes.

3 Beginning at your feet and progressing up to your face, deeply relax your muscles. Keep them relaxed.

4 Breathe through your nose. Become aware

of your breathing. As you breathe out, say the word *one* silently to yourself. Continue the pattern; breathe in… out, *one;* in… out, *one;* and so on. Breathe easily and naturally.

5 Continue for 10 to 20 minutes. You may open your eyes to check the time, but do not use an alarm. When you finish, sit quietly for several minutes, first with your eyes closed and later with your eyes opened. Do not stand up for a few minutes.

6 Do not worry about whether you are successful in achieving a deep level of relaxation. Maintain a passive attitude and permit relaxation to occur at its own pace. When distracting thoughts occur, try to ignore them by not dwelling on them and return to repeating *one*. With practice, the response should come with little effort. Practise the technique once or twice daily but not within two hours of any meal, since the digestive processes seem to interfere with the elicitation of the relaxation response.

Source: R.K. Peters and H. Benson, 'Time out from tension', *Harvard Business Review,* January/February, 1979

Relaxation by numbers – the countdown method

1 Select a comfortable position.

2 Close your eyes, and breathe deeply and rhythmically several times.

3 Take another deep breath and, while exhaling, mentally visualize the number 3. '3' is your symbol for complete body relaxation. (Relax any muscular tension.) Mentally repeat to yourself, '3, complete body relaxation.'

4 Take another deep breath and, while exhaling, mentally visualize the number 2. '2' is your symbol for complete brain and nervous-system relaxation. (Any thoughts, fears, concerns or worries – let them all go. Relax all thought processes, feeling a sense of

mental stillness and harmony.) Mentally repeat to yourself, '2, complete brain and nervous-system relaxation.'

5 Take another deep breath and, while exhaling, mentally visualize the number 1. '1' is your symbol for complete Oneness within yourself, complete mind-body attunement and harmony. Mentally repeat to yourself, '1, Oneness, mind-body harmony.'

6 In this deep state of mind-body relaxation, you are filled with calmness, peacefulness. You are one with the creative forces of your own being, and you may direct these creative forces to bring out positive changes and benefits in your daily life and health. (At this time give yourself any positive health suggestions you wish to hear. If there is a particular part of your body that needs healing, imagine that your own health energies are flowing to that part. Create a tingling sensation, and imagine the body-area bathed in pure light-energy, restoring and renewing every cell and tissue.)

7 When you are ready to continue with your daily activities, say to yourself, 'I have been in a deep, renewing state of mind-body relaxation. I will maintain the perfect attunement I have experienced, and will be in perfect health, feeling better than ever before. I will count from 1 to 5, and at the count of 5 I will feel wide awake and in perfect health.'

8 Then begin counting, '1… 2… 3… 4… 5.' Open your eyes and say out loud (or repeat mentally with your eyes open), 'I am wide awake, in perfect health, feeling better than ever before.'

Source: B.B. Brown, *Stress and the Art of Biofeedback*, Bantam Books, 1977

Relaxation of various parts of your body

1 Select a comfortable place to lie down. Remove your shoes and loosen your belt or light clothing. Stretch out on your back, arms

resting by your sides, feet slightly apart, eyes gently closed.

2 Think to yourself, 'I am now going to relax completely. When I waken I will feel fully refreshed.'

3 Think about your feet, wiggle your toes, flex your ankles. Then 'let go' – let go of all the tension, and let your feet rest limp and heavy.

4 Think of the lower part of your legs, your knees and thighs, up to your hips. Imagine them just sinking into the floor, heavy and relaxed.

5 Now think of your hands. Wiggle your fingers and flex your wrists, then let go – relax.

6 Think of your lower arm, elbow and upper arm, all the way up to your shoulders. Picture all the tension just melting away.

7 Think about your abdomen. Let the tension go, and allow your breathing to flow more smoothly and deeply.

8 Think about your stomach and chest, up to your throat and neck. As you continue breathing more deeply, just imagine all the tension flowing out, and you are relaxing more and more.

9 Now think about your throat, neck and head, feeling limp and relaxed. Relax your facial muscles. Drop the jaw, parting the lips and teeth. Picture yourself completely relaxed.

10 If you are aware of any remaining tension anywhere in the body, go to the area mentally and relax the tension.

11 Continue to remain in this completely relaxed state for five to ten minutes. You may picture pleasant thoughts, or simply blank your mind and enter a stage of light sleep.

12 When you are ready to awaken, say to yourself, 'I have been deeply relaxed. I am now ready to wake up, feeling completely refreshed and relaxed.'

13 Begin to wake up by flexing your ankles and wiggling your toes. Then wiggle your fingers and gently shake your wrists.

14 Bend your right knee and then your left knee. Bend your right arm, then your left arm.

15 Open your eyes. Stretch each arm over your head. Then slowly sit up, stand up, and stretch again. You are ready to continue with your activities.

Source: B.B. Brown, *Stress and the Art of Biofeedback*, Bantam Books, 1977

Progressive Relaxation

This is a three-stage approach to relaxation, focusing on the sources of anxiety, the muscle reactions under stressful or tense conditions, and the continuous practice of muscle-relaxation techniques to control those reactions. Here is the technique in detail:

Since a person generally has very little awareness of the sensation of relaxation, he is asked first to tense a set of muscles as hard as he can until he can feel real tension, even tenderness and pain in the muscles. Then he allows those muscles to relax, and tries to become aware of, to feel internally, the difference between tension and relaxation. For example, in some of the first exercises in Progressive Relaxation the patient is asked to hyperextend the wrist, i.e., to bend the hand so the back of the hand is aiming toward the top of the forearm. The muscles constricting the hand backward are tensed as much as the patient can, and are held until he feels the sensations of tension and even tenderness in the muscles of the upper side and about the middle of the forearm. Then the hand is flopped down to a loose, relaxed position. As a single exercise, this alternation between tensing and relaxing is practised no more than about three times in a fifteen-minute period. A good share of the time is spent in trying to discriminate the feelings of tension and relaxation, i.e., the absence of tension. As practising continues, the patient begins to discriminate more and more finely different degrees of tension and relaxation. The procedure is not hurried; each exercise with each set of muscles is practised for perhaps two weeks, and only then does work begin with another set of muscles. Since the procedure goes progressively through all of the muscles in the body (hence its name), to accomplish the entire procedure requires considerable time, let alone persistence.

Source: B.B. Brown, *Stress and the Art of Biofeedback*, Bantam Books, 1977

The emergency-stop technique
Sometimes things really get on top of you and you need to back off in a hurry before you blow an emotional – or physical – gasket. Here is one method for giving yourself that initial breathing space, that crucial step back to keeping things in perspective. When you are getting worked up:

1 Say 'stop' to yourself.

2 Breathe in deeply and breathe out slowly. As you do so, drop your shoulders and relax your hands.

3 Breathe in deeply again and, as you breathe out, make sure your teeth aren't tightly gritted together.

4 Take two small quiet breaths.

Source: How to Last a Lifetime, Thames Television Limited, 1981

Meditational methods
Meditation techniques vary, but they are all essentially the same in that they aim to develop and exploit inner awareness. It is claimed that, through doing this, exponents can go on to derive a more complete awareness of the outside world, and of their own bodies, and even become perhaps more intellectually efficient as well as physically healthy as a result. Indeed, the best-known meditation technique, transcendental meditation (TM), is described by the TM organization as 'the science of creative intelligence'.

Whatever you are trying, the starting point is a calm, comfortable atmosphere and something

Besides relaxing your mind, meditation techniques can help lower blood pressure.

you can focus your mind on, in order to enter a deep meditative state. TM uses a 'mantra' – a single word or sound given to you by an instructor, whereas other techniques use a single object or idea.

It is indeed relaxing – but will it help you to ward off CHD? Well, certainly many people think that it does.

Studies have shown that during meditation there is a 25 percent decrease in cardiac output, as compared with a 20 percent decrease during sleep, and the heart-rate of the subjects fall by about five beats a minute. Researchers have also found evidence of reductions in blood-pressure. So it seems as if TM may indeed be useful in two ways. First, it induces a soothingly relaxed state of body and frame of mind, which is useful to call upon during highly stressed moments. Second, although this is obviously less clear-cut, it seems to have some direct physiological effects that ought to be beneficial to those prone to coronary heart disease.

On the negative side, I have met people who, while endorsing the benefits of TM, have felt

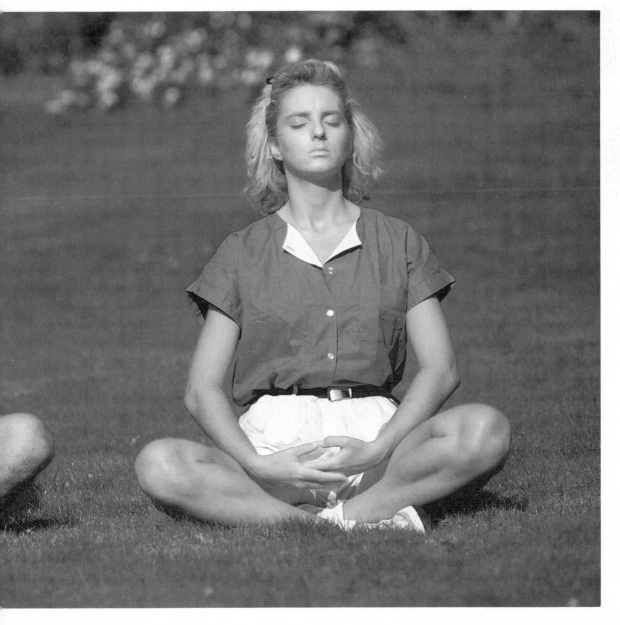

unable to go along with it for any length of time because they felt uneasy about the quasi-religious aspects of the organization. For example, one woman felt, rightly or wrongly, that 'they are trying to get hold of me body and soul'. This may not trouble you at all. Indeed, you may even like the spirituality that bathes the meditational philosophy. At any rate, there is no harm in giving this approach to relaxation a good try.

Biofeedback

If you have trouble relaxing, then a course of biofeedback may be extremely helpful. The idea is to try to use the mind – as in meditation or autogenics (see below) – to control bodily functions in order to influence health. The

Biofeedback technology, giving instant, continuous readings of body functions such as heart-rate.

method has been tried on all sorts of people: headache sufferers, ulcer patients, people with heart arrhythmia, and so on.

What happens is that information about the workings of your own body (the 'bio' part) is fed to you by means of a visual or audio display (the 'feedback'), so that you can see how, say, your heart-rate or blood-pressure is behaving. You then try to exert mental influence over the particular part of your physiology in which you are interested, and, thanks to the instant feedback, you know when you have got the mental 'trick' right and so, after practice, can repeat it more easily in future. There is no magic in this; the body is governed by the nervous system whose chief control centre is the brain. Essentially you are trying to tap into your own control system by conscious effort, rather than simply letting your body systems run freely along their own course.

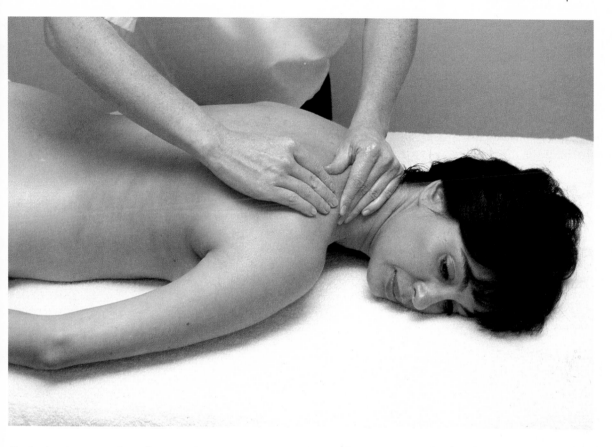

Professional massage. It can just as easily be done by a partner at home.

Biofeedback can be done at home, but it is better to try it under supervision at first. Do not expect miracles; the very fact that you need a machine to help you suggests that this is not a technique for everyday use. Ultimately, the ideal is to control, for example, erring blood-pressure levels without a technological aid, but to date it is impossible to say with scientific certainty whether anyone has achieved this. Think, then, of biofeedback as a support system rather than as a sole means of aiding relaxation – in fact, biofeedback seems to work best in conjunction with other relaxation methods.

Massage and hydrotherapy

While biofeedback machines provide a modern approach to relaxation, massage has been used for centuries to relieve pain, refresh the spirit and calm the body. There are many ways to practice massage, both with a partner and on your own. It is relatively quick, involves no special equipment and greatly helps to reduce built-up tension.

The relaxing effects of water used therapeutically – hydrotherapy – are undeniable. A warm or hot bath, jacuzzi or sauna are all routes to physical well-being. It is a question of trying a variety of methods. Some people prefer the high humidity of a Turkish bath to the dry, hot confines of a sauna. But a word of warning is necessary. Blood-pressure may be reduced in some people after warm baths and saunas, as the body has been plunged into a profoundly calm state of inactivity. But for others – perhaps one in ten – blood-pressure actually increases and so, if you have a heart condition, you should take medical advice before getting too enthusiastic about the joys of hydrotherapy. The question really is: are you feeling better after a spate of intense heat or are you more stressed? If your answer to the latter is 'yes', desist and find another way to relax.

Sauna baths have become increasingly popular for relaxation, especially after a bout of exercise.

Autogenics

Like meditation and biofeedback, this is a method for using the mind to control the body. As with TM, the ideas is to spend 20 minutes a day – perhaps twice a day if you have the time – telling yourself that you feel relaxed, and then focusing on various parts of the body. Say to yourself 'my arm is heavy' or 'my leg is warm', and if the conditions are right you will actually feel that very response. With practice you can focus on other functions such as breathing, heart-rate and so on. To begin with, I suggest you try autogenics with a skilled instructor. To give you some idea of the 'feel' of such a session I have included a transcript of one recorded in an autogenics centre in London.

Many people claim to have found autogenics training – AT – beneficial in the alleviation of their everyday stresses and anxieties, and on that score I see no harm in using it to combat heart disease. As to whether there are any direct physiological payoffs, such as permanently lowered blood-pressure or decreased heart-rate, the evidence is less forthcoming. But autogenics, whatever else, is easy, safe and pleasant, so, if you feel like it, try it.

Sleep

Adequate sleep is vital to health. If you do not get enough high-quality sleep, you feel irritable and under par, devoid of mental and physical energy and enthusiasm.

If you suffer persistent insomnia, your doctor

An autogenics session

Settle back into the autogenic position with your feet flat on the floor, and knees and feet slightly apart. Just rest your arms by the side of you, close your eyes. When you're thinking of warmth you don't have to imagine heat or sun; it's just a very gentle feeling. So if you'd like to focus your attention now inside you, within your own skin, and take up an attitude of mind which is quite casual and passive so that you're not expecting anything to happen... all you're doing is quietly repeating the exercise in your own mind, thinking it through, and I'm going to be repeating it out loud with you. Take your attention along your feet and legs, get to know these different areas in your body, on your legs and back, then to the fingers, hands and arms, taking your attention across your shoulders, and the back of your neck. Think of yourself observing your own body, just quietly acknowledging the different processes taking place, not using your body just now at the moment... don't expect anything to happen but simply acknowledge it as it is; you're your own witness. Let the muscles just flow down your face, including your jaw. Think gently about your right arm, and think the sentence through: my right arm is heavy, then my arms and legs are heavy and warm. Then: my arms and legs are heavy and warm. My arms and legs are heavy and warm. My neck and shoulders are heavy. My neck and shoulders are heavy. My neck and shoulders are heavy. I am at peace. I am at peace. I am at peace. Stay there just for a moment and see how you feel, and then cancel the exercise out by clenching your fists tightly, jerking your arms up to your shoulders to wake you up, take a nice deep breath, and then stretch out, have a good stretch, open your eyes slowly...

Source: Thames Television Limited, transcript of an uncut film from *How to Last a Lifetime,* 1981

may be able to refer you to a sleep clinic for specialist advice. Sleeping tablets are limited in their usefulness, and some even have directly deleterious side-effects, such as raising blood-pressure. If insomnia is only mildly irritating and infrequent, then here is a bedtime routine to get you into the arms of Morpheus.

1 Distract your mind from the problems of the day. Passive TV watching may not do the trick. Better to engross yourself in a book, hobby or conversation.

2 Give your body a change. If your day is mostly spent sitting down, take a walk or do some exercises.

3 Establish a 'getting ready for bed routine', to be carried out unhurriedly and quietly, to slow down your metabolism gradually.

4 Once in bed, find a really comfy position and breathe slowly and gently as if already asleep.

5 Feel the tension draining out of every muscle, starting with your feet and legs and working up through the body.

6 Enjoy the warm heavy sinking sensation that comes over your body. Don't think about going to sleep.

7 Quieten your breathing until it's inaudible and you are quite still. In this state sleep should follow automatically.

If you wake up in the night:

Have pen and paper handy to write down anything that's bothering you. Then you can thankfully sink back into sleep knowing your mind is clear.

If you stay awake:

Don't lie there fretting. Get up, make a hot drink, go back to bed with a book to read until you feel drowsy. Then settle down and go through the routine from stage 4 again.

Source: How to Last a Lifetime, Thames Television Limited, 1981

Chapter 8

How to Stop Smoking:
a plan that works

As a cardiologist I can give you one simple reason for stopping smoking: it will save your life. Studies show that smokers after as little as their first year's abstention have reduced their risk of suffering a heart attack by a full 50 percent. Within five to ten years of quitting, the risks drop to approach those of the nonsmoker. I am not saying that nonsmokers can sit back and never for one moment contemplate the prospect of a heart attack (or, for that matter, any of the other smoking-related diseases), but what is certain is that no other single preventive measure will give you such worthwhile results as spurning the dreaded weed. And, quite apart from health reasons, the benefits of quitting are very great. You will save money, your food will taste better, your complexion will be clearer and your breath sweeter, and you will stop inflicting dangerous smoke on your family and friends.

GIVING UP – AN ACT OF SKILL NOT OF WILL

The big question in your mind, before you get down to the practicalities of giving up smoking, is 'Have I got the willpower?'. You know full well that you are just like the character in Oscar Wilde's play *Lady Windermere's Fan* who confesses: 'I can resist everything except temptation.' You like a puff: it makes you feel good, at least for a while, and it has become a habit, a regular 'fix'.

If, however, you look at people who have been successful in giving up you find that they are not superhuman, but have no more and no less willpower than anyone else. What they do have is a better awareness than others of why they really needed to smoke in the first place. With that knowledge, you can go on to find other ways of fulfilling those needs, ways which do not have the unfortunate adverse medical effects of tobacco products.

Giving up is a matter of knowing why and how you smoke; when a cigarette is needed and for how long. Then you can begin to find alternatives to smoking which will fill the same needs.

Look at the self-analysis chart. Put down your scores in the left-hand column for each type of smoking behaviour – be honest! – and then tally up your scores. If you score 10 or more for any section (perhaps even all), then you can say that this is your 'smoking profile' – the characteristic situation in which tobacco is important for you and to cope with which you will be needing to work hard to find a substitute.

Incidentally, if you do pass the 10 mark in all categories, you must consider yourself as predominantly a 'craver' – someone with a considerable addiction to nicotine which may need a specially designed elimination approach to conquer. I shall deal with this later in the chapter.

HOW, WHY, WHEN AND WHERE?
A THREE-POINT PLAN

Having found out a bit about yourself as a smoker, the next step is to move on to a programme for quitting. You must prepare yourself for this; you are not going to stop today or tomorrow. I suggest you look ahead to, say, a week hence. That will give you time to do three things. First, you can condition yourself mentally to the fact that this is not one of those half-hearted attempts to quit that you have dabbled with a few times before: this is for real and for always. I can hear you now with the

objections and the obstacles: 'Now is a bad time', 'I might succumb to the craving', 'I'll put on too much weight if I succeed'. Put all those quibbles aside for the present and concentrate on the job in hand.

The second reason for looking ahead for a week is so that you can keep a personal 'smoking diary' to note down both the specific times when you smoke and the importance of nicotine on those occasions; I have included an example a good way in which your diary could be set out. This record is going to be extremely important later when you come to ease out of smoking into other activities. Do not forget that you need to keep your chart with you all through the day, and make your notes regularly and systematically.

Thirdly, you need a week to tell other people that you have decided on a set date when you are going to give up. So much of smoking is a social activity: in a pub or club the cigarette is like a token of friendship offered in much the same way as is a conversational gambit. Refusing to accept or offer the token may be regarded almost as an insult. So you have to let people know that, from next week on, you are going to be the same person in every respect except one: you will no longer be taking part in that particular ritual called smoking. Now turn to the 'quitting chart' to get you on the way to stopping and staying that way.

Smoking not only harms the smoker; partners, family and colleagues may also have their health put at risk.

Smoking self-analysis chart

Do you feel like this?	Your smoking type	What's in it for you?
For each statement score as follows: 1 – never, 2 – seldom, 3 – occasionally, 4 – frequently, 5 – always.		
a Smoking a cigarette is pleasant and relaxing ___ b I want a cigarette most when I am comfortable and relaxed ___ c I find cigarettes pleasurable ___ TOTAL: ___	**1 Pleasure/Relaxation**	Most people score highly on this section. Provided you *don't* also score highly on 4, 5 or 6 you are not dependent on the nicotine and should be able to give up fairly easily.
a Handling a cigarette is part of the enjoyment ___ b Part of the enjoyment of smoking comes from the steps I take to light up ___ c When I smoke, part of the enjoyment is watching the smoke as I exhale it ___ TOTAL: ___	**2 Handling**	Fiddling with things is a common way of coping with worries. Everyone has these comfort habits. But if fiddling for you means lighting a cigarette, you should try to find a substitute.
a I light up when I feel angry about something ___ b When I feel uncomfortable or upset I light up ___ c I smoke when I feel blue or want to take my mind off worries ___ TOTAL: ___	**3 Tension**	The more anxious you are, the more you smoke. But smoking keys you up more, it doesn't really reduce tension. Your heartbeat, in fact, speeds up – which may of course direct your attention away from what was making you tense.
a I smoke in order to keep myself from slowing down ___ b I smoke to stimulate me; to perk myself up ___ c I smoke to give myself a lift ___ TOTAL: ___	**4 Stimulation**	Nicotine does stimulate heart-beat and concentration, but by now your body is used to a regular supply and so you need it to feel your 'normal' self. When you give up you won't feel so alert or able to concentrate for a while. It takes three or four weeks to get over this.
a If I run out of cigarettes it is almost unbearable ___ b I am very much aware when I'm not smoking ___ c I get a real gnawing hunger for a cigarette when I haven't smoked for a while ___ TOTAL: ___	**5 Craving**	Do you ever ☐ Drive around late at night looking for a cigarette machine? ☐ Stop work to dash to the shops before closing? ☐ Borrow change to make sure you have the right coins for a vending machine? The craving has got the better of you and you'll have to work hard to beat it.
a I smoke automatically without really being aware of it ___ b I light up without realizing I still have one burning in the ashtray ___ c I've found a cigarette in my mouth and not remembered putting it there ___ TOTAL: ___	**6 Habit**	You may keep yourself so well supplied that you don't have to go long without a cigarette. You may not realize you have a craving for cigarettes. Try keeping yourself in short supply. If smoking really is only a habit you won't feel desperate!

Source: The Open University in association with the Health Education Council and the Scottish Health Education Unit, *The Good Health Guide*, Harper and Row, 1980

THE QUITTING CHART

Giving up	Substitutes	Using your smoker's diary
		If you kept a diary, you can go back to this and tailor your plans to your particular pattern of smoking.
In the two or three weeks before you quit for good, try making smoking less pleasurable: ○ Go and sit somewhere uncomfortable and cold to smoke. ○ Smoke two or three cigarettes quickly and inhale deeply. It feels horrible.	Make an effort and choose to do something else to fill the gap. You should be able to find something else enjoyable to do. In the car, sing along to the radio instead of smoking. Put a record on to relax at home. Carry around something to read when you might smoke.	Did you find you smoked most at coffee and tea breaks, after a meal, with a drink after work, after supper or after you'd made love? These are the key times for which you need to plan definite substitutes for smoking.
Handling something else will probably do the trick. But you need to *plan* to have things to fiddle with.	Do something else with your hands! Keep some scrap paper handy so you can doodle. Fiddle with coins, pencils, paper clips, key rings, jewellery, worrybeads, or special 'executive toys'. Play with a plastic cigarette.	Go through each situation that's linked with smoking for you and plan to do something different. While you're on the phone, shuffle with papers; fiddle with your pen in meetings. Twiddle the lemon in your drink instead of lighting up.
To reduce tension in other ways: ○ Learn a quick relaxation technique and use it! ○ Keep a supply of crunchy foods to bite (carrots are better than hard sweets). ○ When possible go for a brisk walk instead of smoking a cigarette. ○ Ask your doctor for a short course of tranquillizers while you give up.	Try exercises to get rid of anger or frustration. Arm swinging or shadow boxing is effective. Take a brisk walk if you have the time. Learn relaxation exercises so that you can 'let go' instead. Chew something – but watch out! You may substitute eating for smoking.	Are there some things that always make you feel tense? After you've seen your boss? Or an irritating neighbour has called? Plan to run up and down stairs or crunch a hard sweet instead. But as a long-term solution learn how to handle your feelings better.
○ Try waiting until you feel too ill to smoke, then give up at once and completely. You may not need so much 'stimulation' while you're unwell. ○ Your life will seem dull and you may feel less alert at first, so use the money you save to buy yourself 'rewards'.	Buck yourself up with some exercises or a brisk walk, or with a cup of tea or coffee. Turn on your radio to pop music programmes and dance for three or four minutes.	Look at your diary to find the times when you felt most in need of something to buck you up. Plan to do something else instead: make a cup of tea or put the radio or a record on. If you are swamped by pressures at work take time out for a few minutes' relaxation.
○ Don't attempt to give up until you get a smoking-related illness such as a painful cough, breathlessness or heart complaint. ○ Work out really powerful rewards or make a contract to give up for someone you love.	Giving up will be horrible but you will feel so much better once you do manage to stop that you are unlikely to want to smoke again. You may have started smoking very heavily when you had a lot of problems. You may need to get help for these problems rather than risk going back to smoking or substituting alcohol or pills.	Because the nicotine level in your blood is low you will feel a real craving for the first cigarette of the day. But don't be tempted to give up slowly by cutting down instead of cutting out. It prolongs the agony. During the withdrawal symptoms keep reminding yourself that you knew you would feel like this and that you are proud of yourself for giving up.
Before you quit for good make yourself aware of when you want to light up so that you don't later on find yourself smoking without realizing it: ○ Keep your pack in a different pocket; leave your lighter in another room. ○ Watch for trigger events, like using the telephone or having a cup of coffee, when you tend to light up automatically.	You don't need to replace this kind of habit. Watch out you don't start popping sweets into your mouth unnoticed instead!	Keeping the diary going may help you give up! Having to make a note each time you smoke makes you aware of how much of a hold the habit has on you.

Nicotine addiction

Most smokers have an element of nicotine dependency in their habit. As your body begins to lose traces of nicotine the cigarette craving begins, and then you begin to experience the nicotine withdrawal symptoms. You become irritable and anxious. You begin to wonder whether you might not be far better off unhealthily happy than miserably fighting fit.

There are two ways you can help matters. The first is *not* to stop all at once, but to go through an initial period of cutting down (as distinct from trying to give up by 'tailing off' your smoking, a method which almost never works); this is not ideal, but the fewer you smoke the better. Although it is frequently said that the only way to give up smoking for good is to stop abruptly and altogether, this is often extremely difficult – especially if you smoke more than a pack a day. Instant 'cold turkey' is not always best. So, if you find that you simply cannot stop smoking right now, try to cut down in the following ways:

Remember that the unburned part of the cigarette acts as a filter. If you can put the cigarette out before it is half-smoked, you will avoid taking in a significant amount of toxic material.

Don't inhale. If you do, don't inhale deeply.

Ration yourself and stick to the ration. Make sure you smoke fewer than 15 a day – any more and soon you will be back to a pack a day.

Try a pipe or cigars instead of cigarettes, and don't inhale.

Smoke the lowest-tar cigarette available.

If you smoke a pipe or cigar, ration yourself. Use filters. If you're a pipe-smoker, use less tobacco; if a cigar-smoker, buy smaller cigars.

Concentrate on one of the 'trigger' situations at a time. For instance, to start with give up smoking after meals. Once you have managed this, go on to the next trigger. Treat yourself to something as a reward for progress. Have a

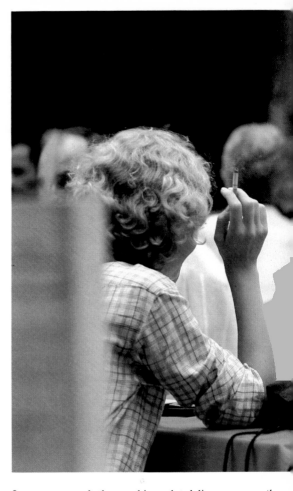

Lung cancer and other smoking-related diseases are on the increase in women.

definite timespan in mind for stopping completely – don't make it too protracted or your enthusiasm and willpower may wane.

If even this proves hard, work out the times of day or situations when you most need to smoke and allow yourself to do so then, but only then.

Source: M. Polunin (Ed.) *The Health and Fitness Handbook,* Windward and Here's Health, 1981

Strategy number two is gradually to reduce the amount of nicotine in your tobacco intake. You smoke *the same number of cigarettes* (this is most important) but over a four-week period you

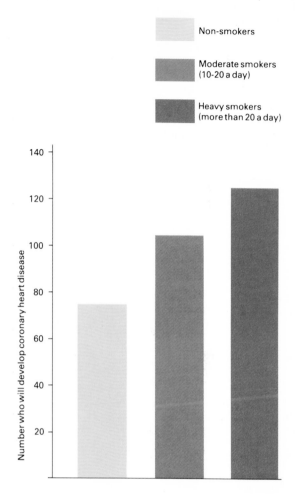

- Non-smokers
- Moderate smokers (10-20 a day)
- Heavy smokers (more than 20 a day)

Number who will develop coronary heart disease

Out of every 1000 men aged 40 to 60 years, the number who will develop CHD is strongly affected by the number of cigarettes smoked per day.

gradually switch to a low-tar brand so that you end up adjusted to far lower levels of nicotine. At the end of the four weeks you can then have a stab at quitting altogether, and your 'cold turkey' will have less shattering effects. It is often easier to give up than to stay off cigarettes for good; many people achieve abstinence for a few months and then revert to cigarettes for one of many reasons, like a personal crisis or a holiday period. See the section on relapse, below. And, above all, don't be too disheartened if you don't manage to give up the first time. It may take several attempts.

The day you stop smoking
The big day comes. How do you feel? You may feel in a bad mood, nausea and stomach upsets may plague you, perhaps you will find yourself coughing more than usual as your lungs begin to function without toxic smoke swirling around

deep inside them. One thing you must not do is just sit there feeling miserable. Practice what psychologists call a 'displacement activity'. Take the morning off if you can, and do something quite out of the normal routine. In fact, try to make sure you avoid routine altogether. If you look back over your diary you will see how your smoking habits are very closely linked to routine, so break the mould. Do not lie in bed twitching for a cigarette, but get up early and wash the car or clean a few pairs of shoes. Keep a bunch of keys or a string of beads by the bed where the packet used to be and fiddle with those instead. Remember that a lot of the oral pleasure of smoking can be derived instead from drinking a glass of orange juice or sucking a mint. Try it.

A SMOKER'S DIARY

When you smoked	Fri	Sat	Sun	Mon	Tues	Wed	Thur	3	2	1	0
First thing – in bed	—	—	—	—	—	—	—	—	—	—	—
Getting up	—	—	—	—	—	—	—	—	—	—	—
At breakfast	—	—	—	—	—	—	—	—	—	—	—
Travelling to work	—	—	—	—	—	—	—	—	—	—	—
Starting work	—	—	—	—	—	—	—	—	—	—	—
When a problem came up	—	—	—	—	—	—	—	—	—	—	—
Answering the telephone	—	—	—	—	—	—	—	—	—	—	—
In the bathroom	—	—	—	—	—	—	—	—	—	—	—
At tea/coffee break	—	—	—	—	—	—	—	—	—	—	—
With a meal (except breakfast)	—	—	—	—	—	—	—	—	—	—	—
After a meal	—	—	—	—	—	—	—	—	—	—	—
Waiting to meet someone	—	—	—	—	—	—	—	—	—	—	—
Over a drink	—	—	—	—	—	—	—	—	—	—	—
While driving	—	—	—	—	—	—	—	—	—	—	—
While reading	—	—	—	—	—	—	—	—	—	—	—
Doing the housework	—	—	—	—	—	—	—	—	—	—	—
At the shops	—	—	—	—	—	—	—	—	—	—	—
At the pub	—	—	—	—	—	—	—	—	—	—	—
Watching TV	—	—	—	—	—	—	—	—	—	—	—
Last thing at night	—	—	—	—	—	—	—	—	—	—	—
After making love	—	—	—	—	—	—	—	—	—	—	—
Other times	—	—	—	—	—	—	—	—	—	—	—

Column groups: **How many smoked** (Fri–Thur); **General importance ratings** (3 2 1 0)

TOTAL SMOKED

How to score on the importance ratings:

3 if you were desperate for a smoke

2 keen

1 just felt like it

0 didn't realize you were lighting up

Source: The Open University in association with the Health Education Council and the Scottish Health Education Unit, *The Good Health Guide,* Harper and Row, 1980

Actually, many ex-smokers, when questioned, say that they experienced hardly any ill-effects at all: it amazed them how easy it was.

Staying off cigarettes

The first day – or even week or month – may turn out to be quite easy. But what about the long years ahead? How can you remain an ex-smoker?

One strategy to help you stay stopped is to build some kind of incentive scheme into the whole business of changing your habits. You might, for example, enter into an anti-smoking pact with another smoker so that you reinforce each other's determination.

Here is a five-point plan to help you stay stopped:

1 The first six to twelve months are the most critical period. You must remain on guard during that time. Afterwards you will have a far greater degree of control.

2 Avoid situations that are stressful or anger-making, or better still have an armoury of anti-stress measures such as one of the relaxation techniques described in Chapter 7 ready to use at crisis points.

3 Don't fool yourself that you can try just one cigarette without being hooked, or that you

Many people smoke more under stress. Making the workplace a no-smoking area can help people give up.

should have one for old time's sake. Don't use tenuous rationalizations such as 'smoking will keep my weight down'. If you are overweight, try a safer method of slimming.

4 Spoil yourself by reminding yourself how much healthier, wealthier and self-disciplined you have become. To kick a long-term habit is some achievement, so glory in it from time to time!

5 You may wish to try anti-smoking aids such as nicotine gum (this should be done under medical advice) or anti-smoking self-help groups. You could also try acupuncture, if you feel like experimenting with something exotic, or hypnotism (making sure that the practitioner is properly qualified). Anti-smoking clinics run by health departments also exist in some areas.

Relapse

No one is superhuman. You may well lapse back into the habit. This is not unusual, and it does not mean that you are a failure – or that you cannot get on the right road again. Do not feel guilty, as this causes anxiety which in turn may well reinforce the smoking behaviour. Think of your temporary lapse as just an isolated event that you will put behind you. It is a question of picking yourself up, dusting yourself off and starting all over again, with another attempt at the anti-smoking programme. Take it again from the top.

Chapter 9
Diet and Keeping Fit

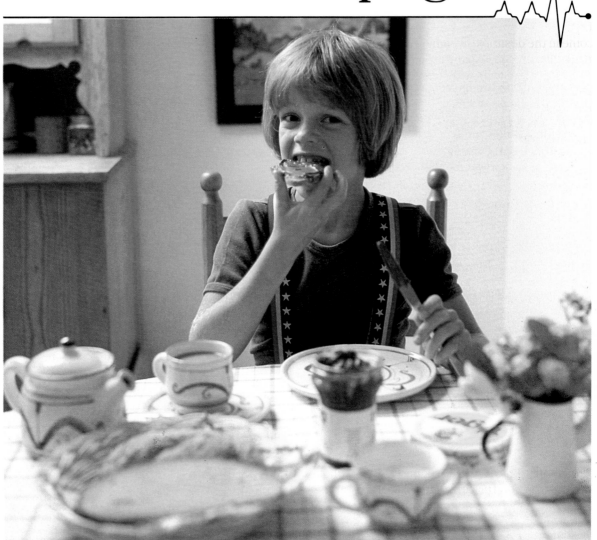

LOSING WEIGHT – IT CAN BE DONE

You do not have to have a medical degree to know that excess weight is bad for the cardiovascular system, or that it can increase the risk of other diseases. That said, there are no hard and fast rules to govern any individual's particular body-shape: there is no simple correlation between being overweight and getting ill. However, the available evidence very much supports the view that excess weight is physiologically and psychologically a bad idea.

Walking round an art gallery recently, I was struck by the way in which our image of what is physically desirable has changed so much over the centuries. Today, small is beautiful, slim is healthy, lean is attractive. We find our sexual idols not in the indolence of luxuriant aristocratic life, with its Rubensian plumpness, but out on the running track or tennis courts; not consuming great mountains of pheasant and exotic spices but lunching on salad followed by a yoghurt and an apple.

CAUSES OF OBESITY

Look at the guidance charts and see where you come in the desirable-weight scale. Anywhere to the right of 'acceptable' and you will want to try to make a few changes to move yourself to the left. But what has caused your excess fatness in the first instance? Well, there are a lot of misconceptions flying around, old wives' tales and just plain self-defence mechanisms fogging the picture.

Patients come to me saying that they are fat because their parents are or were fat. It is, they argue helplessly, genetic. It runs in the family. And they will often take out a family snapshot to prove the point.

Scientific research in recent years has undermined the inheritance idea. No doubt fat parents tend to have overweight children, and there are many fat people who seem to put on weight excessively by eating only a little, as if they had some inbuilt metabolic aberration dictated by their genes. But far more pertinent, in my view, is the fact that children are brought up in an environment determined by their parents' behaviour. The chubby baby is often the baby to whom too much food is given. He or she grows up learning fat-making eating habits, fat ways of cooking and fat attitudes to food. Thus, while I do not rule out a genetic component in regulating the way we store up body-fat, I most put this in second place, behind bad eating habits.

Most children love junk food, but adults should encourage a balanced diet if they are to help their children to avoid becoming fat adults.

Are you overweight?

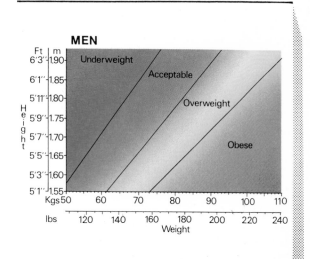

Eating self-analysis questionnaire

Answer the questions below as accurately and honestly as possible, using the following code:
1 – never, 2 – rarely, 3 – sometimes, 4 – usually, 5 – always. Place the number in the box next to the statement.

1   I skip breakfast. ☐

2   I have a snack or nibble when watching TV. ☐

3   I have a snack or nibble when preparing meals. ☐

4   I eat sensibly in front of others and splurge when alone. ☐

5   I eat when I am unhappy. ☐

6   I eat in response to physical hunger sensations. ☐

7   Meals in restaurants or in other people's homes make me eat more than I should. ☐

8   I eat more at weekends than during the week. ☐

9   I eat more than usual when I am on holiday or vacation. ☐

10   I wake up in the middle of the night and eat. ☐

11   I eat more and more as the day goes on, once I begin to overeat. ☐

12   I have an uncontrollable urge to eat even to the point of making myself sick. ☐

TYPE ONE:

Externally controlled eating

The relevant questions here are numbers 1, 2, 3, 6, 7, 8, 13, 16, 19, 22, 26, 27, 35 and 37.

Question 1 4 or 5 scores 1. Several studies have shown that 79 percent of overweight people say they skip breakfast, as compared to 44 percent of normal-weight people. The uneaten calories are often made up later in the day. It is better to eat more calories at breakfast than at dinner. Better distribution of calories throughout the day equals better diet control and less overeating.

Questions 2 and 3 4 or 5 scores 1. Preparing food and watching television are very strong eating cues for many people. They make people want to eat even when they are not hungry. Also, eating while involved in something else such as reading makes you less aware of how much you are eating.

Question 6 1 or 2 scores 1. Many externally controlled overweight people do not seem to respond mainly to hunger sensations; they eat because they cannot help being 'turned on' by food cues around them.

Question 7 4 or 5 scores 1. People who are very susceptible to the sight or smell of food find the attractive presentation of food in a restaurant or in someone's home especially stimulating.

Question 8 4 or 5 scores 1. During the week, mealtimes are usually fairly routine, dictated by the hours spent at work. But weekend leisure-time offers more opportunities. People used to eating by the clock still eat at their usual mealtimes, but also when they see friends. Socializing at weekends becomes associated with drinking and eating.

Question 13 1 or 2 scores 1. A very common feeling. Conscious resistance to external cues has broken down. Guilt arises from knowing that the external cues are stronger than one's efforts to resist them.

Question 16 4 or 5 scores 1. People easily tempted by food tend to want it without delay. So they stand up while eating, nibbling a bit of this and a bit of that, without feeling full as they would after eating a proper meal.

Question 19 4 or 5 scores 1. Many overeaters use the clock to tell them when to eat. Time also influences how much they eat. Deliberately setting a clock to the wrong time can affect the amount they eat. When the clock says 'lunchtime' – even in mid-morning – they often hunger for their usual lunch.

Questions 22 and 26 4 or 5 scores 1. The sight of food has a huge influence on the eating habits of externally responsive eaters, as does plentiful food within easy reach. Food is seldom left untouched or unfinished. If small portions are given and second helpings are not on view or not offered, less food can satisfy them.

13   I feel guilty after I have eaten a lot. ☐

14   When I lose weight, I can control my emotions better. ☐

15   Eating keeps me feeling better emotionally. ☐

16   I eat standing up. ☐

17   I eat food even when it doesn't taste very good. ☐

18   I think about and look forward to each meal. ☐

19   The time of day influences my eating. ☐

20   I consciously restrain my eating, or else I overeat. ☐

21   I overeat when I'm angry or depressed. ☐

22   I eat when I'm not really hungry, just because food is available. ☐

23   When I am bored I eat for something to do. ☐

24   My body just seems to crave food. ☐

25   I'm willing to make a special trip to the shops or prepare something to satisfy my cravings. ☐

26   I finish whatever is put in front of me. ☐

27   When small meals are put in front of me, I feel satisfied and don't want second helpings. ☐

Question 27 4 or 5 scores 1. When food cues are weak, many sight-and-smell eaters find it relatively easy to go without eating, sometimes making do with less than people who are not externally responsive. Even total abstinence is possible, provided food cues are removed. One study found that when fasting was part of a religious ritual, externally responsive overeaters found it easier than normal eaters – as long as they stayed away from all external food cues.

Questions 35 and 37 4 or 5 scores 1. The smell of food is a powerful stimulus for eating, to which the externally cued person can hardly fail to respond. The sight of other people eating has much the same effect – whether or not the person is really hungry.

So, for this part of the questionnaire, the maximum score is 14. If your score is 10 or over, consider yourself an externally controlled eater.

TYPE TWO:

Emotionally cued eating

The relevant questions here are numbers 5, 14, 15, 17, 21, 23, 32, 40 and 41.

Questions 5 and 21 4 or 5 scores 1. Many people eat in response to emotions, usually anxiety or anger. For a few people, feeling happy is a more likely signal for overeating. Possibly our emotions weaken our defences against overeating or arouse us to find food more attractive.

Question 14 4 or 5 scores 1. Feeling good because you're in control of your eating reinforces your determination not to eat.

Questions 15, 23 and 40 4 or 5 scores 1. Overeating is a common response to anger and unhappiness even in normal-weight individuals. So it is important for you to know whether eating is a *satisfying* response to your problems.

Question 17 4 or 5 scores 1. If you eat to make you feel less unhappy, then even food that doesn't taste good may have the desired effect. If you think you might be 'rewarding' yourself in this way, try to assess the true taste of the food you are eating before you eat too much.

Question 32 4 or 5 scores 1. If food is a very important factor in your life, you will feel *emotionally* deprived when food is rationed or withdrawn. Hence the success of flexible weight-loss programmes which help people develop substitute rewards.

Question 41 4 or 5 scores 1. People who 'live to eat' tend to think of food as a source of emotional pleasure. This is not to say overeaters are emotionally disturbed: eating in response to emotions is not a sign of disturbance *per se*. But it may indicate that you tend to use food as a substitute for other pleasures, or to reward yourself too often with food.

If you have given yourself 5 or more out of

Eating self-analysis questionnaire continued

28   I overeat when I drink alcohol. □

29   I'm likely to eat too much if I'm doing something else at the same time (watching TV, reading, talking). □

30   When I diet, I get more headaches. □

31   When the afternoon comes, my stomach rumbles. □

32   When I don't eat (or when I'm dieting), I become nervous and anxious. □

33   I think about food when I am not actually eating or preparing it. □

34   I feel dizzy and faint when I go without food. □

35   The smell of good food is an irresistible temptation to start eating. □

36   It is easier to control my eating in a restaurant than at home. □

37   Other people's bad eating habits (at home or work) make me eat the things I shouldn't. □

38   I eat most when I have already eaten a lot. □

39   I do better on diets which specify exactly what and how much to eat than on diets which leave me more choice. □

40   When I eat because I have problems, eating makes me feel better. □

41   Food is one of my major satisfactions. □

a possible 9 points for this section, you eat for emotional reasons.

TYPE THREE:
Internally cued eating

The relevant questions here are numbers 1, 5, 6, 8, 10, 12, 21, 22, 24, 25, 30, 31 and 34. Internally cued and externally cued eating are, to a large extent, two sides of the same coin. So some of the questions relevant to external cues turn up again here.

Questions 1 and 8   1 or 2 scores 1. If you seldom or never skip breakfast, it is because you generally wake up feeling hungry. Also the physical signals which prompt you to eat are the same no matter what day of the week it is.

Questions 5 and 21   1 or 2 scores 1. Feeling miserable, nervous or worried can arise from increased sugar in the blood, which generally stops internally controlled eaters from eating. If you are

one of them, you will not eat, let alone overeat, when you feel unhappy.

Question 6   4 or 5 scores 1. Responding to every physical sensation of hunger is the big give-away for all internally cued eaters.

Question 10   4 or 5 scores 1. 'Night starvation' may be due to not eating enough during the day; the physical sensation of hunger may be strong enough to wake you.

Question 12   4 or 5 scores 1. Feeling full to the point of nausea usually stops anyone eating. It is *needed* only when earlier signals are not working properly. A controlled eater anticipates fullness and stops eating before feeling sick.

Question 22   1 or 2 scores 1. Food on display or easily available is not a turn-on to internally cued eaters.

Questions 24 and 25   4 or 5 scores 1. A strong craving for food and preparedness

to make an effort to get it are both good indicators of internally controlled responses. Food craving increases the more you deprive yourself of food. If you crave specific foods, you may have a deficit of some particular nutrient.

Questions 30, 31 and 34   4 or 5 scores 1. Headaches, dizziness and a growling stomach are all signs of hunger – low energy reserves.

If you scored 10 or more out of a possible 13 points on this section, you can consider yourself an internally cued eater.

TYPE FOUR:
Consciously restrained eating

The relevant questions here are numbers 4, 9, 11, 13, 18, 20, 28, 29, 33, 36, 38, 39. A consciously restrained eater who is overweight is something of a paradox. Self-restraint and overeating appear to be mutually contradictory. The problem is

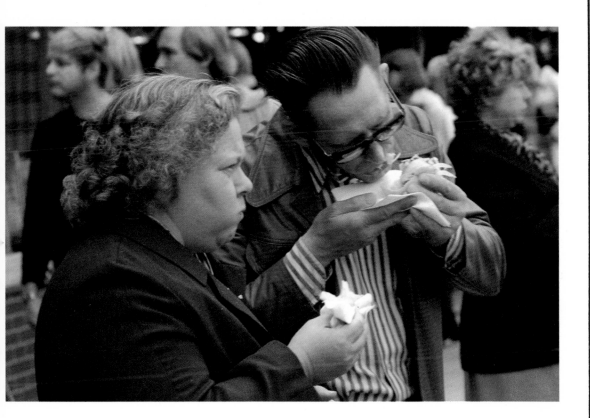

that self-restraint is easily disrupted – by strong emotions, by distraction, by alcohol consumption, and so on. Continuous, focused attention on *not* eating too much, being negative, is difficult to maintain.

Questions 4 and 13   4 or 5 scores 1. If you feel very guilty about eating, you are probably not exercising as much control over your eating as you would like. Eating in secret does the most damage to your self-respect. To achieve permanent weight control, you must overcome your guilt.

Question 20   4 or 5 scores 1. There are many fat and formerly fat people who control their weight by being consciously aware of their desire to eat. They feel very tempted by food, but they consciously fight the desire to eat.

Questions 9, 11 and 38   4 or 5 scores 1. Consciously restrained eaters really let go when they stop monitoring themselves. As the nursery rhyme goes: 'When she

was good, she was very, very good, but when she was bad, she was horrid.'

Questions 18 and 33   4 or 5 scores 1. Thinking about food and looking forward to meals occasionally indicate physiological deprivation; more usually they are a sign of conscious control of eating.

Questions 28 and 29   4 or 5 scores 1. Overeating is most likely when you are distracted from your conscious effort to restrain yourself. Restraint is a flimsy mechanism precisely because it is so difficult to maintain. And once you have overeaten your motivation to keep fighting takes a big knock. Many people overeat hugely once their restraint breaks down.

Question 36   4 or 5 scores 1. For the consciously restrained eater, eating in a restaurant is less dangerous than eating at home – portions are controllable, and second helpings usually out of the question.

Question 39   4 or 5 scores 1. A wide choice of menu stimulates the appetite and puts a great strain on self-control. This is why most consciously restrained eaters prefer diets which allow them next to no choice. On the other hand, regimes which involve more choice and decision-making are more successful in the long term, because they are closer to real-life situations, and so less easily broken.

If you scored 9 or more out of a possible 12 points on this section, you can consider yourself a consciously restrained eater.

Source: J. Rodin, *Controlling Your Weight,* Century, 1983

194

Do not, as many people also tend to do, attribute your weight to 'big bones' or 'glands'. Tests show that obese people, within the limits of normality, have completely regular bone structure. They do not need to carry great amounts of fat on them. Nor do they have bizarre glandular disorders. Less than one in 200 people may have an underfunctioning thyroid gland, but by-and-large the glandular story is a red herring.

Another explanation for fatness is that fat people are excessively lazy and inactive. Again, there is confusion here. It is true that fatter people tend to be lethargic – but is this the cause of the fatness or an effect of it? It could be the latter. Furthermore, in modern urban society the majority of people lead a fairly sedentary existence; for many of us our daily exercise consists of walking to the car, from there to the office and on to the canteen, and at the end of the day driving home again for an armchair evening in front of the television. But not everyone who lives like this is overweight.

Nor should you subscribe to what I call the emotional-retribution theory of fatness: that people are overweight because they are anxious, inadequate, self-indulgent or neurotic. The vast majority of overweight people are psychologically well balanced. Some fat individuals may well

These two men are of regular height and build, but differ enormously in weight.

be depressed by their fatness, but once again this is more likely to be an effect than a cause.

Inappropriate eating

People are overweight because they eat too much of the wrong sorts of foods, while at the same time failing to expend sufficient calories through physical activity to burn off the input. Later in this chapter I shall deal with the right sort of foods to aim for, with the kinds of exercises that are appropriate for maintaining a proper 'energy budget'. Here, though, I want to dwell on *why* people eat too much. If you are overweight, identifying the cause(s) is the essential first step to losing weight and also to *staying* slim.

HOW DO YOU EAT?

What sort of eater are you? We all have a pattern of eating keyed-in to our lifestyle. If we are overweight, then somewhere along the line we have to see just what is wrong with that pattern. The first step, as in the anti-smoking programme, is to keep a diary so that you can find out how much you eat, when you eat it and why. You should keep the diary for a week or two, making sure that those weeks are fairly typical and not out-of-the-ordinary periods, such as holidays. You need to note down all the times you eat and drink, including extra snacks between meals; how long you spend at meals and snacks, nibbling extras; where you eat and whether alone or with others; in what moods – neutral, morose, excited; and whether or not you are actually hungry on each occasion.

Once you have done this you will be in a better position to fill in the *eating self-analysis questionnaire*. This is designed to identify the sort of eater you are. This knowledge can then be used effectively in a reducing regime.

ANALYSING THE QUESTIONNAIRE RESULTS

According to Dr. Judith Rodin, who devised the eating self-analysis questionnaire, there are four types of eating that will emerge from your scores: 'externally controlled', 'emotionally cued', 'internally cued' and 'consciously restrained'; further details are given below. If you have worked through the questionnaire with the aid of your diary, you will probably find that you score high on one of these types, possibly two. From there you can go on to find a personal tailor-made strategy for improvement.

AN ACTION PLAN

Beating externally controlled eating

Obviously the problem with this type of eater is that he or she lives in a world full of food-related cues, ranging from chocolate advertisements on street hoardings to fixed-point ritual dinners with parents-in-law. Breaking the pattern is not going to be easy. How, for example, do you get round the fact that you are the type of eater who gets 'hungry' the second the clock reaches a notional – or indeed official – lunchtime? One approach is consciously to decide not to eat lunch at exactly

A typical supermarket offering a vast range of foods. There is a growing trend to display Calorie content and nutrition details on food packages.

the same time each day, or to skip a mid-morning snack altogether – not because these measures will in themselves cause you to shed pounds, but because they will lead to that all-important dissociation between stimulus and response. Similarly, you might try to cut out all eating in front of the TV, or munching sweets behind your desk, or whatever. Avoid the sight and smell of food as much as possible. Make detours to avoid the odours wafting out from that French bakery. Go into the kitchen as little as possible, making sure that anything you might want during the day is elsewhere.

Beating emotionally cued eating

In much the same vein, you should try to interpose something between yourself and an emotional cut to eating. If you feel that food is for 'comfort' or 'pleasure', then it must follow that, at those times of acute susceptibility, you need to find substitutes – or better still, attempt to prevent the need to assuage strong feelings in the first place. Try to get to the root of your anxiety or preoccupation and work on that.

Beating internally cued eating

The approach here is much the same as for externally cued eating. Look for ways of preventing automatic responses to every sensation of 'hunger'. Try to reshape lifetime habits by changing long-established mealtime routines.

If you are a food-craver type who seems driven by the body to get satisfaction, you will have severe difficulties in overcoming the urge. It is very hard to argue with hunger pangs on the grounds that they are 'conditioned' by one's timetable. This is where an eating technique might be of use. Taste every mouthful s-l-o-w-l-y – not necessarily cutting down on quantity to begin with, but learning to appreciate everything you taste. Take small mouthfuls. When you begin to feel you have eaten enough, get into the habit of leaving some food on your plate – none of that mother-knows-best non-sense of finishing up good food to the last crumb.

Beating consciously restrained eating

From the questionnaire analysis you can see that the secret here is self-awareness. It is particularly useful for you to keep up your daily

diary, because you are the type of eater who can exercise considerable control provided you are operating within a strict framework. Watch, too, for events and situations that will undermine your authority over yourself, like parties, eating out and travelling. Your main worry is that you might switch from control to chaos after a sudden lapse. Try to remind yourself that, as with smoking, one deviation does not mean that you are an inferior being, nor that you will never get back on the right lines again.

WEIGHT-LOSS AIDS

What we have been discussing as a means of self-management is really a form of behaviour therapy. You are trying to change long-assumed internal or external conditions that seem always to produce a certain response. In your case, that response is eating, and it is possible to get help with this. You may consult a clinical psychologist specializing in behavioural methods, or perhaps enrol in a relaxation class to find ways of damping down the emotions or anxieties that lead to overeating.

There are also prescribed drugs to help reduce weight, but these are used only in extreme cases. The same is true of surgery.

Eating habits, not genetic factors, result in fat families.

A typical high-fat, high-calorie meal.

The increasingly popular fruit and cereal breakfast with a minimum amount of fat is just as filling and quicker to prepare.

Some very obese patients have part of the small intestine removed, thereby reducing the amount of their food-intake that their bodies can absorb. Dental splinting is an even more extreme remedy, involving the wiring up of the jaw to prevent eating anything unless it's in a liquidized form. Sometimes doctors recommend starvation for short periods to get weight off quickly. But remember that you should never contemplate taking these measures without prior medical advice.

More often you will find it useful to enrol with a self-help group, such as Weightwatchers. Such groups can make you put your own fatness problem, if problem it is, into some kind of perspective by comparing it with other people's. Do not waste your money on over-the-counter drugs which claim miraculous effects overnight.

But my most important single piece of advice is to *stop thinking of yourself as a lifelong dieter*. You are not. You are eating perfectly well. You are not depriving yourself. All you are doing is changing the nature of your eating patterns in a small way to keep your weight to a desirable level. It is just good sense replacing anarchy.

EATING YOUR HEART OUT

Millions of words have been written on the vexed subject of diet and heart disease. To the observer – the doctor as well as the patient – these endless attempts to understand how our diet may or may not cause atherosclerosis, high blood-pressure or high cholesterol levels have resulted in a tangled skein of dos and don'ts. We all want to avoid a coronary – for the first or second time – but with the best will in the world we just do not know how to set about it. Is fibre the answer, for example? Should we eat saturated or unsaturated fats? And, while we are at it, should we become vegetarian or vegan to prolong our lives?

In fact, there is no absolutely right path for anyone and everyone. So what I want to do here (and the same applies to exercise) is to admit the limitations of any specific, detailed eating schedule (we are not farm animals, after all) and instead offer the basic principles on which to base your own personal regime.

The aim of the dietary programme is to eat

Just a few of the vegetables which can make up healthy, and also colourful, meals and snacks.

prudently, which means adopting a regime designed around what we already know about the relationship of food to heart disease.

Aim for a balanced diet. You should eat a mixture of foods – and have a reasonably controlled intake of food. Cut down on those fattening items that the body can easily do without, such as sugar and sugary foods, alcohol, fatty foods (especially animal and dairy produce), and processed carbohydrates.

Reduce your intake of fats, saturated and unsaturated. Avoid butter, margarine, cooking fats and oils (cut right down on fried food), cheese, cream, fatty meat (cut fat from meat before cooking), pastry, cake, crisps, nuts, rich sauces or soups, salad dressing and mayonnaise.

Eat less salt. Salt can aggravate hypertension – see Chapter 5. Sodium chloride, common salt, is found in many foods, especially processed packages. A single hamburger, for example, probably contains as much as or more than the body needs for its daily intake.

Forget the idea of 'dieting'. If you eat along the lines I am suggesting, then you will eat both sensibly and adequately, with great enjoyment. To maintain a healthy heart you do not have to subject yourself and your taste buds to some rigid assault course.

ACQUAINT YOURSELF WITH FOOD

You should get to know food in a biochemical way because, the better you understand what you put into your body each day, the more you will appreciate its effects on the cardiovascular system.

Carbohydrates

Found in starchy and sugary foods, carbohydrates are an easily digested source of short-term energy; marathon runners, for example, binge on pasta for a day or longer before a race. Low-carbohydrate diets used to be fashionable for slimming, but now it is recognized that, for slimming and for general health, fats and high-protein animal produce, which form an increasing part of the average diet in affluent societies, should be cut down, and carbohydrates, especially those high in fibre, increased. Examples of good carbohydrate sources include wholemeal bread, pasta, rice, peas, beans, lentils and potatoes – the staple starchy foods which used to comprise a big proportion of the diets of the poor.

Fibre

As people have become in general more affluent, they have begun to eat a higher proportion of processed foods and meat and other animal products, and less of the staple carbohydrate-rich foods – although the idea that fibre is good for you has been catching on fast in recent years. Claims have been made that plenty of fibre in the diet helps protect against a number of ailments, from constipation to heart disease, by increasing the bulk of indigestible matter passing through the gut, thereby improving and speeding up its action. It is possible to keep slim on a high-fibre diet: taken at the expense of rich, processed food, fibre can help cut down your intake of high-calorie foods by filling you up more satisfyingly. You don't have to become a vegetarian, and you will find that foods like wholemeal pasta can be made into a wide variety of delicious dishes.

There are two main groups of fibre-rich foods. The first includes cereal foods made from whole grain, like bread made from wholemeal flour, bran-based breakfast cereals, brown-rice dishes, and wholemeal pasta, biscuits and crackers; ordinary brown bread and ordinary pasta also contain some fibre – you don't have to exclude the less fibrous starchy foods completely. The other type of fibre is found in the undigestible cellulose – the roughage – of fruits and vegetables. These make a very important contribution to any diet, especially if, where possible, you eat also the skins of fruits and potatoes and the green leaves – preferably raw – of vegetables like spinach, cabbage and cauliflower. Among the vegetables the pulses – such as peas, beans and lentils – also contain lots of protein.

Proteins

These are the essential 'building-block' foods. By contrast with the richer, primary protein sources like red meat and eggs, which are also high in fats, vegetable and cereal sources of protein, such as beans, peas, lentils, soya protein and wholemeal bread, are doubly good because they are rich in fibre. Fish and chicken are good sources of low-fat animal protein, and it has also been suggested that fish has a beneficial effect on lowering blood cholesterol.

Fats

You will probably be familiar with the controversy that has been raging in recent years over the sort of fatty foods that are considered dangerous to the heart and blood vessels. In case you are not familiar with it, however, the argument goes as follows. *Saturated* fats, which are primarily of animal origin, as in meat and eggs, are known to be associated with the deposition of cholesterol plaque within blood vessels. This, it has been claimed by some researchers, is incontrovertible – while the effects of *unsaturated* fats (many, but not all, vegetable oils) have not been proven to be dangerous: in other words, cook with sunflower or soya-bean oil rather than lard or butter and you will be less susceptible to atherosclerosis.

The great danger is that many people now assume that unsaturated-fat consumption is healthy. It is not. A recent Norwegian study of likely ways of reducing heart disease came to the conclusion that the best way to minimize your risks is to cut down on *all* fats, of whatever kind!

Some way of cutting your fat intake may seem fairly obvious, such as trimming the fat off meat before cooking or eating. Others are less well known. For instance, there is more fat absorbed by French fries (chips) if they are crinkle-cut than if they are straight cut, because the crinkles increase the surface area. For the same reason, thick French fries are better than thin ones.

PREPARING FOOD

The way in which you prepare and serve food is also important: for example, as we have just noted, straight French fries cut in large pieces are preferable to the smaller crinkled variety.

It is now well known that the various types of Oriental cooking are among the world's healthiest cuisines.

And try to leave the skins on! People also tend automatically to serve food doused in butter or dressing, thus adding more fats *and* calories to the meal. With a little more thought and experimentation – for instance, using herbs and spices in cookery – the flavour of food may be enhanced without all this extra fat.

As a general rule, grill instead of fry.

Frying should be done only with vegetable oils like pure sunflower or olive oil. Never use lard or products labelled simply 'vegetable oil'.

Roast meats in foil instead of basting them with fat. Try to cut down on roasts; boil, stew or grill meat rather than roast it in its own fat.

Make gravy from the sediment left *after* the fat has been drained off the meat – but cut down on meat-based gravies in general.

Make sure cooking oil is hot enough before adding food, as otherwise excessive fat will be absorbed. Have the occasional stir-fry, Chinese-style; this is a much healthier and tastier way to eat fried food.

Non-stick pans are preferable because they need little or no oil.

Use a liberal amount of kitchen paper to absorb surface fats on all foods before they are eaten.

This wide range of foods comprise much of what is needed for a varied and satisfying diet. Note how many foods are high in fibre.

How about alcohol?

A drink or two a day, it appears, may inhibit the aggregation of protective platelet cells around the damaged walls of an artery, thereby reducing the chances of a clot forming or of a constriction growing to impair blood-flow. But the hazards of alcohol in excess are almost too well known to need spelling out: it causes dependence, all kinds of physical debilities, deaths from drunken driving and domestic accidents, poverty, disrupted relationships, and crime. These hazards occur when consumption has reached a 'problem' level. Most patients ask: will my usual couple of drinks a day damage my heart? In general the answer is no: in fact, alcohol in moderation – say a glass of wine at lunchtime and another in the evening – is positively beneficial. But any more than this is a bad idea for all sorts of reasons, one of the main ones being that alcohol is high in calories and is thus very fattening.

EXERCISE AND THE HEART

Generally speaking, all parts of the body which have a function, if used in moderation and exercised in labours in which each is accustomed, thereby become healthy, well developed and age more slowly; but if left unused and idle they become liable to disease, defective in growth and age quickly. (Hippocrates, 300BC)

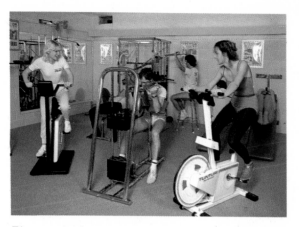

Fitness enthusiasts enjoying a session in the gym. You can keep fit without having to set aside time every day or use special exercise equipment.

I had two good friends, both cardiologists, who died suddenly within months of each other. They were both jogging at the time. (Christiaan Barnard, AD1984)

The heart, like all other muscles, can be trained to perform better and be stronger and more reliable. What is more, should it become weakened by a heart attack, it can be re-trained back up to a level approaching pre-infarct fitness. There is now evidence showing that some of the established risk factors in CHD – namely elevated cholesterol levels, high blood-pressure, intolerance to sugar and a tendency to rapid blood-clotting – are all actually decreased by suitable physical-training routines.

In practice, this means that exercise can have quite dramatic effects in improving the health of your heart. A study carried out on 17 000 students from Harvard University showed clearly that, within certain limits (see below), the greater the amount of regular physical activity the subjects underwent, the less likely they were, all other things being equal, to suffer a first heart attack. If the subjects burned up an extra two to three thousand calories a week through exercise, a marked decline in infarcts resulted. Interestingly enough, this same study showed that, when subjects took more exercise than this, it did not appear to reduce their chances of getting a heart attack any more than for those burning up just an extra two to three thousand calories, demonstrating that a modest but regular amount of exercise – say, a few kilometres' walking, swimming or maybe running, five days a week – is all that is required for limiting the risk of cardiovascular disease.

Cooking vegetables in a wok ensures that vitamins are not lost.

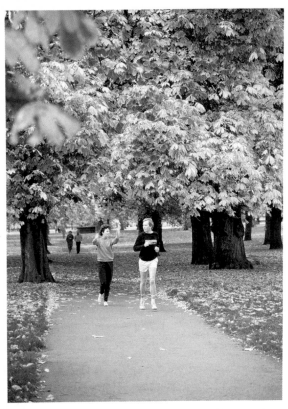

A brisk walk or jog is excellent exercise and relieves tension – best done away from heavy traffic and car fumes.

Swimming in particular is an excellent form of safe exercise for the heart and every other muscle in the body – as well as being most enjoyable.

How much is enough?

The findings of the Harvard study bear out other investigations performed elsewhere.

First, it is good sense to exercise on a *regular* basis: the most dangerous thing you can do – and the dangers increase in direct proportion to your age – is to rouse yourself from a state of total inactivity (such as a week at the office) to a sudden hour or two of violent activity on the squash court. Training any muscle is a steady, cumulative process, not an exercise in masochistic over-activity.

Secondly, you do not need to do very much exercise at all to meet the requirements of a health-promoting regime. No need, in short, to let your whole life be dominated by an obsessive urge to sweat and strain every available minute of every day. Sufficient exercise can be taken within the context of an ordinary busy life, and there is no need to drop other things in order to timetable it.

Choices of activity

Anything you do that gives you some form of regular, unstressful activity will benefit your heart: if you can combine this with enjoyment, then so much the better. In fact, never choose an activity just because it is 'good for you': you will soon get bored of it. Watch the streets of London, New York or any other city during the week following a marathon. They will be alive to the sight and sound of joggers puffing round in imitation of the heroes they saw completing the 26 mile 385 yard course on television. But how many of these new enthusiasts will continue to jog throughout the long winter evenings in rain and snow? Very few, because running, especially solo, simply does not suit everyone. Indeed, most people prefer their sporting activities to include a little social interaction and competition, such as you get from badminton.

Also, never feel that it *has* to hurt to be beneficial. By all means work up a good sweat, and even perhaps a thirst for a well deserved glass of beer. But do not push too hard. Tune-in to the warning signals from your body. If you are puffing frantically, feeling any chest pains or dizziness, or finding it difficult to recover from a bout of exercise, then you are doing the wrong thing. Consult your doctor. The most beneficial

Exercise alone is not enough to reduce large amounts of unwanted flesh – you have to cut down the Calories too.

forms of exercise for the heart are those that build up stamina – the aerobic forms of exercise.

Aerobic and non-aerobic exercise

Ever since Jane Fonda's programme of aerobic exercises hit the market, people have been singing the praises of aerobic exercise as if it were some new method of activity. Cardiologists, however, have long known that aerobic exercise produces beneficial effects on the cardiovascular system.

The word 'aerobic' simply means 'requiring oxygen', and refers to exercise which requires oxygen to be delivered to the muscles. Anaerobic exercises, by contrast, are those where oxygen-supply is not required or available. For example, if you take a brisk walk or a gentle jog, you are exercising aerobically; your heart pumps blood containing oxygen and other essential nutrients to all the muscles involved. Suppose now that you went into a sudden hard sprint, putting high energy demands on the cardiovascular system. For a time it can keep up with these demands, but after a while the heart's pumping ability and the muscles' capacity to extract energy are pushed to their 'anaerobic threshold'. At that point the energy to keep the muscles working comes, not from the supply of fresh oxygen, but from energy resources which are already stored within them. Because these energy resources are limited, you very quickly tire. Compare the champion sprinter, who is exhausted after ten seconds or so, with the marathon runner, who keeps going for over two hours, or even longer.

For cardiac health, we should be concentrating on aerobic exercises to build up oxygen-giving efficiency. We are looking also for continuous or 'dynamic' exercises, like walking, cycling and swimming, rather than explosive, strength-endowing but largely stationary activities such as weight-lifting or water-skiing.

Sometimes a compromise is desirable or inevitable. Golf and baseball, for example, are not particularly helpful to the cardiovascular system because they are not continuous and dynamic. However, a gentle set or two of tennis is preferable to nothing at all, while a round of golf – provided you do not linger too long over the nineteenth hole – will at least get you

Regular exercise is most pleasurable when it is part of your life's routine. If you're not used to strenuous exercise, walk-don't-run should be your motto at first.

walking. And don't get too frustrated if you consistently lose: exercise should give you relief from stress, not *more* competitive tensions!

Compromises occur in other ways, too. Cycling provides excellent exercise; like swimming, its intensity can be adjusted to suit your own level of fitness and performance – it is a perfect self-regulating activity, always at the right pitch for the individual. However, riding a bike in cities can be dangerous. If cycling is what you want to do, you may have to confine your exercise to weekends in the park together, perhaps, with mid-week 'excursions' on an exercise bike at home or in a gym.

When choosing a method of exercise that might suit, bear these general guidelines in mind:

1 You should consult your doctor before embarking on any strenuous exercise programme if you are over 30 or if you have had heart trouble or any other physical problem which could be aggravated by overdoing it. Jogging, especially, should be done in moderation.

2 If exercise makes you gasp for breath or causes you pain, stop immediately – and talk to your doctor about a modified programme.

3 Try to get 20 to 30 minutes of continuous exercise a day, or at least every other day. Supplement formal exercise with everyday surrogates, such as walking up flights of stairs rather than using an elevator.

Swimming is one of the best forms of continuous, dynamic exercise that can be enjoyed by people of all ages and fitness levels.

The solitude of the lone runner.

Some sporting activities do not necessarily tone up heart and lungs, but they do relieve stress and get you out of doors.

4 Keep at it. You should be thinking that your regular exercise is here to stay... and so, in the process, are you!

SAFE TO START EXERCISE

Before embarking on any exercise programme you should test how fit you are already. A simple and safe way of doing this is to measure your pulse rate. The first thing you want to know is the rate while the body is at rest, so the measurement should be taken first thing in the morning before the rate can be affected by exertion, tension, nicotine, coffee, tea or alcohol. Rates vary, but 70 to 85 beats per minute is the average for men and 75 to 90 beats is the average for women – generally speaking, the slower the pulse the fitter the person.

Whatever your sex, if your resting pulse rate is in the nineties you are unfit, and if it is over 100 you have cause for concern and should seek an immediate check-up. Once you have established that you are reasonably fit, you must check on the safe maximum pulse rates you can achieve during exercise.

Even without taking your pulse, it is easy to get an idea of how fit you are by completing the

How to take your own pulse

What you are actually feeling when you take your pulse is the waves of blood travelling from the heart along a main artery. The pulse is normally felt at the wrist, because the beat is strong and in an easily accessible place, but pulses can be felt in many other parts of the body, such as the neck.

To take your pulse, use a watch that shows seconds. As shown, hold the watch in your left hand and hold the left wrist with your right hand – move the first two fingers of your right hand until you can feel the pulse just under your thumb on the left wrist. Count the number of beats that occur during a thirty second interval and then multiply by two to get

the number of beats per minute. To get the 'resting pulse' you should do this first thing in the morning, while you are sitting in a relaxed position.

The next step is to work out what your safe maximum pulse rate during exercise should be. This depends on two things: your age and your current level of fitness. For a fit person, the heart can beat at a maximum of about 200 beats per minute at age 20, but at only about 150 beats at age 70. When you are exerting yourself, your pulse rate should not rise about 75 percent of your maximum. A useful and very safe formula for calculating the ideal rate for you is: 200 minus your age minus another 40 if you are very unfit. Thus for an unfit 50-year-old the rate would be: 200–50–40 = 110 beats/minute.

The graph gives you an at a glance estimate of the approximate desirable rates during exercise for different ages and levels of fitness.

checklist below. Put a tick in the box for yes and a cross for no.

I can feel my heart thumping after climbing a few flights of stairs. ☐

I am left gasping for breath even if I run only a short distance. ☐

It is a terrible effort to bend and tie my shoelace. ☐

I ache all over digging only a small patch of the garden. ☐

I am tired out after moving the lawn with a hand-mower. ☐

I am tired out after carrying two bags of shopping for a quarter of a mile. ☐

I avoid physical effort if I possibly can. ☐

If you have ticked any of the above and are aged under 50 years, you probably would benefit from more exercise.

There follows a series of exercises which you can do in the home which will increase general fitness and make you strong and supple.

The following exercises can be fitted into the pattern of your daily life; you don't need to change into sports clothes, use special equipment or travel to the local gym. They are not intended to strengthen any particular part of the body, but they will make you more flexible, less tense, and are a good starting point for embarking on a special exercise programme.

As a general, very important rule, take exercise whenever you can. Walk or cycle instead of taking the car – you will sometimes even find this quicker for moderate distances. Walk upstairs where possible. Housework and gardening are good ways of ensuring that you get

GENTLE EXERCISE

Put hands on shoulders and move your elbows up and around, making circles.

Climbing stairs two at a time is a good, energetic form of exercise for strengthening hip joints and thighs as well as heart and lungs.

regular, gentle exercise. You can even incorporate some floor exercises into sedentary pastimes like watching television; indeed, if you spend much of your day sitting, you should stand up and walk about at regular intervals. The body should not be kept in the same position for long periods, so alternate one kind of activity with a totally different one. Although mild forms of exertion may not seem to have any effect on your strength or your waistline at first, remember that something as basic as walking a few miles a week *every* week will provide long-term well-being and, of course, will help to keep your weight down.

To give the upper spine a good stretch after sitting for a long time, clasp your hands, palms facing outwards. Round your back, tuck your chin in, and push your hands outwards, stretching your arms away from you.

Lie facing up with your arms straight out by your sides, palms down. Prop your legs on a low stool or box. Push your hips as far as you can in comfort, and hold the position for a few seconds.

To strengthen the upper back, prop folded arms on a high surface, thus raising your shoulders.

When standing, for example during a telephone call, raise yourself up and down on your feet. This strengthens and improves circulation in the calves and feet.

You can do this exercise for stretching the lower back sitting on the floor, standing up or lying down. Bend one leg up and clasp it tightly, then the other leg.

Lift your leg out to the side and put it on a desk. This gently stretches the hips and inside leg so it should not hurt. Lift each leg up in front of you to stretch the backs of the legs.

BASIC DAILY WORK-OUT

Hold out your arms to shoulder height and
move them backwards in small circles, with
elbows kept straight.

With feet apart and bottom tucked in,
stretch upwards as far as you can, breathing
in deeply, and keeping your head up. Try
this in a doorway, so that you stretch
upwards towards the frame.

Stand in front of a wall and move forward
slowly so that your palms are placed against
it. Keeping your body straight, breathe out
and lean further forwards, bending your
arms. Then breathe in and push yourself
away from the wall by straightening your
arms.

A well-known exercise for heart and lungs
is stepping on and off a chair. Move slightly
forwards and step up onto the chair with the
left leg then the right, straightening up with
both feet together. Then step down, left leg
then right, and straighten up.

Chest and shoulders
a) Stand with your arms stretched out, with your fists clenched.
b) Breathe in, then breathe out and swing both arms in a strong sweep across your chest and then outwards, breathing in.
c) Repeat the action, swing the arms across in front of your face then bringing them down in front of your hips.

Arms

a) Raise your arms so that they make a right angle at shoulder level.

b) Turn your forearms so that your hands point downwards, maintaining the right angle at the elbow, pressing your hands backwards, then relax. Try this only once or twice at first.

Abdomen

a) Sit on the front of a chair with your legs straight out and heels on the floor. Lean back gripping the sides of the chair and bend both knees, bringing your thighs up against the body.

b) Once you can do this with knees bent, try it without bending your legs.

Abdomen and back

a) Kneel on all fours, and looking upwards, breathe in deeply and arch the centre of your back downwards.

b) Breathing out, tuck your head in and curve the centre of your back upwards with your tummy muscles tucked in.

Legs

Stand behind a chair, holding on to the back. Squat down. then come back up on your toes, straightening your legs. Then repeat. This squatting exercise makes many people realise how seldom they bend their knees other than for sitting.

Bottom and hips
a) Lie down with your arms out to the sides, palms downwards.
b) Bend your left leg upwards and bring it down across your body without lifting your shoulders.
c) Raise your leg to the centre and bring it down out to the side. Bring it back to the centre and slide the leg straight out ready to start again with the other leg.

TWO AEROBIC EXERCISES TO KEEP THINGS TICKING OVER

Skipping
Easily done at home, this popular exercise increases the pulse rate and more oxygen has to be taken in and carried through the body. Skip until you are panting comfortably (around 50 to 100 skips should do it).

Jogging

This is one of the most popular forms of
keeping fit. You should take great care
when you start jogging, remembering to
alternate it with walking.

NEVER TOO LATE

Ask a pessimist how much wine he has in his glass and he will say that it is 'Half empty'. Ask the optimist the same question and the reply is 'Half full'. I find that people have these two opposing attitudes to their own health, especially the health of their heart. There are those who take the view that, whatever they do – be this a change in diet or lifestyle, or both – there is no changing The Way They Are. If they are destined to have a coronary in middle life, then so be it. It is probably, they say, written in my genes anyway so who am I to rewrite Nature?

Other people adopt a more positive approach. They are willing to try anything, change their ways, attempt to take control of things, to beat the enemy. And these are the people who do not complain that they are too old for remedial or preventive measures to do any good.

You will, I am sure, know from this book what my own attitude is. One is never too old to improve one's health. True you may have passed your whole life so far unthinkingly consuming a high cholesterol diet. Or puffed away relentlessly on a couple of packs of cigarettes daily. But you *can* make a fresh start and, if you do, this will – and I stress this strongly – be reflected in a healthier heart: one that will carry on doing its job for you longer than it would have done had you not taken action.

No one can achieve immortality, but we can, using the knowledge provided by science blended with common sense, live a healthier and longer life. More than that, we can also have that incomparable feeling of being in control of our own destinies. Working positively for good health, as opposed to passively hoping, is a tonic in itself. And from what I said earlier about the nature of stress, you will appreciate that this very feeling of holding the reins is itself a useful weapon to combat heart disease.

Index

Page numbers in *italics* refer to relevant captions

A

aerobic exercise 203
acyanotic tetralogy 60
adrenalin 85, 90, 137, 142, *157*, 158
Akutsu, Tetsuko 46
alcohol (drinking) *49*, 52, 122, 141, 143, 155, 200
ambulatory monitoring 147
anaerobic exercise 203
anaesthesia 26
anastomosis 27, 105
Andreason, Anthony 32
aneurysm 101-102
angina 24, 66, 70-71, *70*, 84, 90, *94*, 97, 121; recurrent 130, 136; sex and 135
angiogeneisis 148
angiograms *80*
angioplasty 149-50
angiotensin-converting enzyme inhibitors 143
antibiotics 25, 103, 110
antibodies 110; monoclonal 145, *146*
anticoagulants 92, *92*, 101; oral 92
anti-foam 35
antithymocyte globulin 111
aorta 18, 19, 62; anastomosis 105; aneurysm of 102; coarctation of 62
aortic arch *17*
aortic stenosis *59*
aortic valve *see* valves
apex beat 73-4
Aristotle 12-13
arrhythmias 25-6, 94, *94*, 122, 148; in foetus 53; *see also* heartbeat (abnormalities)
arteries 19, *19*, *24*; blocked 86, 99; cleaning 150; coronary 23, 24, 86, 90, 96-9, 121; diseases 23-4, 146; hardening *see* arteriosclerosis; pulmonary *17*, 18, 19, 62; *see also* aorta; atherosclerosis; coronary-artery disease
arteriography 103, 130
arteriosclerosis (hardening of the arteries) 23, 24, *65*, 66, *66*
ascorbic acid (Vitamin C) 95
aspirin *92*
asthma 71, 91, *91*
AT *see* autogenics
atheroma 23, *24*, 66, 103, 138
atherosclerosis 66, 83, 92, 99, 138, 147, 199
atresia 62

atria *17*, 18, 19, 58, 128
atrial flutter 76, *77*
atrial septal defects *see* septal defects
atrio-ventricular block 26
atrio-ventricular node 23, *23*
atropine 128
auscultation 74; immediate 73
autogenics (AT) 176, 178, 179
autonomic nervous system 90, 94
azathiaprine 111

B

bacterial endocarditis 60
bacterial infections 99, 103
Bain, Donald 147
balloon angioplasty 140-50
balloon pumps 150-51
balloon valvutoplasty 150
Barnard, Christiaan *passim*, *et* 7, 33-5, *34*, 37, 40-43, 96, 101, 201
Benson, Herbert 170
beta blockers 90-91, 94, 142, 143
Betaloc (metoprolol) *91*
beta receptors 90
bezafibrate 92
Bigelow, Wilfred 29
Billroth, C.A. Theodor 14
biochips 118
bioengineering 44-6
biofeedback 176-7, *176*
Björk–Shilley valve 99
Black, Mrs 42
Blaiberg, Philip 42-3, *44*
Blalock, Alfred 27-8
blood 19, 20, *20*; 'blue' 19
blood cells: red 20, 86; white (leukocytes) 20; *see also* platelets
blood circulation 18, *18*, 19, 20, 27; pulmonary 55, 56; systemic 55
blood-flow, rate of 24
blood groups *20*, 40
blood pressure 20, 85, *137*, 149, *174*, 177, 179; diastolic 138, 139, 140, 143; high *see* hypertension; measuring 138-40, 143; systolic 138, 139-40, 158
blood transfusion *20*
blood vessels: synthetic 44; walls 148; *see also* arteries; capillaries; veins
'blue babies' 27-8, *27*, 32, 34, 56, 59-61, 111, 148
Boerhaave, Hermann 13
Bond, Gene 147
bradycardia 26
breathing disorders 89
breathlessness 71, 136, 142
Breckenridge, A.M. 148

bretylium 94
Broken Heart, The (Lynch) 87
bronchitis 71, 85, 103
Brunton, Lauder 15
bubble oxygenator 35, *37*
bypass operations *see* coronary-bypass surgery; heart surgery

C

calcification 99, 101
calcium blockers 143, 148-9
cancer 85, 144; lung 71, 85, *184*
capillaries 19, *19*, 20
carbohydrates 198
carbon monoxide 85-6
cardiac asthma 71
cardiac glycosides 89
cardiomyopathies 24
cardioplegic solutions 102, 104
cardio-pulmonary (heart) resuscitation 123, 124-5
Carrel, Alexis 40
catheters, cardiac 40, *41*, 76-8, *78*
cells *146*
cerebral haemorrhage *see* stroke
CHD *see* coronary heart disease
chest pains 70-71, 141, 142; *see also* angina
chlorothiazide 90
cholesterol 66, 82, 92, 95, 122, *146*, 199, 201; diets to lower 83-4; drugs to lower 84-5
cholestyramine 84, 92
cigarettes *see* smoking
circulation *see* blood circulation
Clark, Barney 115, *115*, *116*, 150
clonidine 143
cloning 145
clots (thromboses) *20*, 24, 66, *67*, 86, 92, 146, 148, 200
clotting 86, 145, 201; prevention 33, 92, 94
CMV 146, *146*
coarctation 62
coffee 85
congenital disorders: causes 50; heart 26, 27, 48-63, 65, 148; multiple 62-3; obstructions 59; valves 25, 59, 99
consciously restrained eating 192-3, 194-5, 196
contrast radiography 78
convalescence *see* heart attacks (aftermath)
Cooley, Denton 41, 46
cooling for surgery (hypothermia) 29-31, *29*, *30*, 32, 34-5
Cooper, Prof. Cary 170
coronary arteriograms 130

coronary artery *see* arteries
coronary-artery disease 23-4, 66, 136; surgery for 96-9
coronary-artery grafting 130
coronary-bypass surgery 96-9, *96*, *98*, *149*; *see also* heart surgery
coronary care units 127-9, *128*, *129*
coronary heart disease (CHD) 65, 69; death-rates 69, 86-7, 119, 144; family histories of 82; genetic influences on 145; incidence *69*, 137, *185*, 201; male-female susceptibility differences 87; symptoms 69-72
coronary occlusion *80*
coronary sinus *17*
coronary thrombosis *see* thrombosis
corticosteroids 111
coughing 71, 142
coumarin 92
Coxsackie viruses 24
cramps 142
cross-circulation 32-3, 34, 35
Culpeper, Nicholas 89
Cutler, Levine and Beck 16
cyanosis 60, 148; *see also* 'blue babies'
cyanotic congenital heart disease *see* 'blue babies'
cyclophosphamide 111
Cyclosporin-A 44, 111
cystic fibrosis 71
cytomegalovirus (CMV) 146, *146*
cytotoxic antibodies 110

D

Darvall, Denise 42
DeBakey, Michael *44*, 96
defibrillation 119, 122, *122*, 126-7, 128
demand pacemakers 118
Demikhov, Vladimir 40, *41*
dental splinting 197
depression 141
desopyramide 94, 128
De Vries, William *46*, 115, *150*
De Wall, Richard 35
diabetes 50, 82, 91, 102, 103
diagnosis 37-40, 44, 52, 69-80, 96, 122, 146-7, *147*
diamorphine 113
diastolic pressure *see* blood pressure
diet 155, 188-200; balanced *189*, 198; deficiencies of 71; hypertension and 140; imbalances of 155, 194; improvement 131, *134*, 142; *see also* diets; eating habits
diets 95, 135-6; low-cholesterol 83-4; reduced-fat 84, 136; starvation 197; *see also* obesity
digitalis 89-90, *89*, 147
digitoxin 89
digoxin 89, *94*
diuretics 90, 93-4, 142-3
dizziness 141, 142
DNA *145*
Dogliotti, Achille *63*
donor availability *see* heart transplants
Doppler ultrasound 147

drinking *see* alcohol
drinking-water *see* water
driving 135
dropsy 89
drugs: anti-atherosclerosis 92; anti-heart-failure 88-95; anti-rejection 44; cholesterol-lowering 84-5; heart transplants and 103; hypertension and 142-3; pregnancy and *49*, 51-2, 91; recently developed 146, 147-9; selection of 95; weight-reducing 196; *see also* anticoagulants; immunosuppressives; side-effects
ductus arteriosus 148; *see also* patent ductus arteriosus

E

eating habits 190-93, 194-6, *196*; *see also* diet
ECG (EKG) *39*, 74-6, *76*, *77*, 105, 113, 121-2, 147; exercise 75, *75*
echocardiography *see* ultrasound scanning
edema *see* oedema
effort syndrome 71
Einthoven, Willem *39*
Eisenmenger's Syndrome 56, 111
EKG *see* ECG
electrocardiography *see* ECG
embolisms 92
emotionally cued eating 191-2, 194, 195
emphysema 71, 103
endarterectomy 99
endocarditis 25, 60
energy budgets 194
enzyme inhibitors 143
epicardial implantation 118
epicardium 118
E-type 148
exercise *132*, 136, 142, 143, 155, 194, 200-217, *202*, *203*; aerobic 203; anaerobic 203; regularity of 202, *203*; starting 204-205
exercise ECGs 75, *75*
exercise tests 75, 130-32, 135
exhaustion curve 158
externally controlled eating 190-91, 194, 195

F

fainting 71
Fallot, É.-L.-A. 59, 60; *see also* Tetralogy of Fallot
fats 84, 92, 136, 197, 198, 199
fetal heart *see* foetal heart
fibre 198, *200*
fibrillation 31, 110; atrial 26, 76, *77*; ventricular 76, *77*, 126, 136
fibrin *20*
fibrosis 101; cystic 71
fight-or-flight response 156, 158
film oxygenator 32
first aid (after heart attack) 122-7
Fisher, Hans *95*
fixed-rate pacemakers 118
Fluon 44

foetal heart *see* heart (prenatal development): pregnancy
Fonda, Jane 203
food *see* diet
Forssman, Werner 39-40, 76-8
foxgloves 89, *94*
Framingham study 80-83, 85
Friedmann, Meyer 166

G

Galen 13, 20, 26
Garrett, Edward 96
genes 165, 145
genetic engineering 145
German measles 50-51
Gibbon, John 31-2, 35
Gibbon's oxygenator 32
glucose intolerance (sugar intolerance) 82, 201; *see also* diabetes
glyceryl trinitrate 90
glycosides 89
Gott, Vincent 33-4
grafting 59
Gross, Robert 26-7
guanethidine 143

H

haemoglobin 20, 86
haemorrhage 113; cerebral *see* stroke
Hales, Stephen 139
Hardy, James D. 41-2
Harvey, William 20, 40
headaches 141
heart: artificial *44*, 46, *46*, 113-17, *113*, *116*, *117*, *149*, 150, *150*; historical ideas about 11, 12-18; modern research on 144-51; muscle *17*, 23-4, 59, 136; parts of *17*; prenatal development 48-53, *52*, 55, 80; pumping action 22, 23; rhythm *see* heartbeat; shape 18; size 18; stress and 158-9; workings 18-23; wounds to 13, *13*, 15-16; *see also succeeding entries*
heart attacks (infarcts) 66; *77*, 84, 120-43, 146-7, 161; aftermath of 99, 118, 130-36, *130*, 148; first aid after 122-7; incidence 159, 180; recurrence of 136; vitamins and 95; *see also* coronary heart disease; myocardial infarction
heartbeat 22, 85, 117, 118, 119, 149; abnormalities 71, 75-6, 94, 128; apex 73-4; new-born child's *55*; regulation of 19, 23, 25-6; slowing 29, 90-91, 128-9; *see also* arrhythmias; bradycardia; pulse; tachycardia
heart block, complete 128-9
heart disease 23-6; acquired 64-119, 155; 'alternative' treatments for 94-5; causes 80-87; congenital *see* congenital disorders; coronary *see* coronary heart disease; costs of 82; family histories of 122; ischemic *see* ischemic heart disease; preventing 155-218; rheumatic 25; surgery for 96-102 (*see also* heart surgery); treating 88-119; viral 24
heart failure 71, 72; drugs to combat

88-95, 148; left 71; right 71
heart–lung machines 31, 33-4, *38*, 40, *56*, 58, 107, 110, 149; *see also* lungs (artificial); oxygenators
heart–lung transplants 56, 111
heart murmurs 74
heart-rate 158; *see also* heartbeat; pulse
heart resuscitation *see* cardio-pulmonary resuscitation
heart stimulants 103
heart surgery 13, *14*, *15*, 26-46, 52, *56*, 60-62, *61*, 63, 96-102, *100*; bypass 27-8, *32*, 58, 59, 84, *97*, 101, *149*; closed 28; coronary-bypass 96-9, *96*, *98*, *149*; history of 14-18, 26-37; mortality rates 97, 99; valve *see* valves; *see also* heart transplants
heart transplants 34, 40-44, 46, 94, 102-111, *104*, *105*; aftercare 110, 111-13; animal 40; care of donor heart 103; donor availability 40, 41-2, 102, 103, 104; first 7, 15, 37, 42, 115; heterotopic ('piggy back') 110; patient selection for 102-103
hemoglobin *see* haemoglobin
hemorrhage *see* haemorrhage
heparin 92
hepatitis B 103
heredity 140, 145
heroin 113
heterotopic transplants 110
hibernation 29, *31*
Hine, Lily 16
Hippocrates 12, 73, 200
His, Bundle of 23, *24*, 26
HLA 110
holes in the heart *see* septal defects
Holmes, T. 160, 161-2
Holmes Sellors, Thomas 28
Holter, Norman 147
hormones 85, 90, 137, 158; hormonal abnormalities 140
Hufnagel, Charles A. 44-6
human leukocyte antigens 110
Hume, R. 95
hydrotherapy 177
hypertension (high blood pressure) 82, 83, 103, 122, 148, 158, 198, 201; causes 140-41, 159; countering 136-43, 170; primary 140; secondary 140; symptoms 141-2, *142*
hypertrophy 82
hypothermia *see* cooling for surgery
hypothyroidism 50

I

immunology 145-6; *see also* rejection
immunosuppressives 40-41, 42, 103, 110, 111, 112
incompetence, valve 25
Inderal (propanolol) *91*
indigestion 70-71
infarcts *see* heart attacks; myocardial infarction
inferior vena cava *17*
inflammatory disorders 146

influenza 51
insomnia *see* sleep
internally cued eating 192, 194, 196
intragastric cooling 34-5
ischemia 24, 130
ischemic heart disease 96, 148, 150
Ivalon 44

J

Jarvik, Robert 46
Jarvik-7 artificial heart *116*
job stress *see* work
junk food 155, *189*; *see also* processed food
Justus, Wilhelm 14, 15

K

Kantrowitz, Adrian 150-51
kidneys 93-4, 103, 113; disorders 140, 143; failure 136; transplants 40-41, 42
Kilb, Dr. 46
Kiss of Life 124
Klebanhoff, Gerald 44

L

Laënnec, René 73
Lanoxin (digoxin) *94*
Larrey, Dominique-Jean 13
laser artery cleaning 150
LDL-C 84
leukocytes 20
Lewis, John 29, 33
lifestyle 65, 69, *69*, 135-6, 142
lignocaine 94, 128
Lillehei, Walton 32, 33, 34
lipids *65*, 85, 92, *146*; metabolism 145
liver 103
loneliness 87
Low Density Lipoprotein–Cholesterol 84
Lowe, James 70
lungs 19, 31, 35, 55-6, 113, 149; artificial 31; cancer 71, 85, *184*; flooding 56, 58; *see also* heart–lung machines
lymphocytes 112
Lynch, James 86-7

M

Maclean, Una 134
Magill, Ivan 26
massage 177, *177*; heart 15
meditation 170, 174-6, *174*; transcendental (TM) 170, 174-5, 178
Melnick, Joseph 146
membrane oxygenator 35-7
memory lapses 142
methyldopa drugs 142
Meuffels, Willebrordus 46
Milrinone 147-8
mitral stenosis *see* stenosis
mitral valve *see* valves
monitoring techniques 37-40, 147, 151
monoclonal antibodies 145, *146*
morphine 113
mouth-to-mouth resuscitation 124

myocardial infaction *80*, 121
myocardial ischemia *see* ischemic heart disease
myocarditis 146
myocardium 23, *24*, 148

N

Navidrex-K *93*
neoplastic conditions 48
nervousness 141
nervous system, autonomic 90, 94
nervous system, cardiac 23, *23*; defects of 25-6
nicotine 85, 86; addiction 181, 184-5
nicotinic acid 92
nicoumalone 92
nitrates 90
nitrites 90
nitroglycerine 90
Nixon, Peter 158
NMR 147
noradrenalin 142
normotensive readings 139-40
nuclear magnetic resonance 147
nutrition *see* diet

O

obesity (overweight) 66, 71, 82, 86, 140, 142; causes 189-94; control 131, 136, 143, 155, 189-9; 'inherited' 189, *196*; surgery and 196-7
oedema (edema) 71, 89, 142, *142*
open-heart surgery *see* heart surgery
operations *see* heart surgery
Osler, William 69
overweight *see* obesity
oxygenators 31-2, *33*, 35-7; *see also* heart–lung machines

P

pacemakers: artificial 26, *26*, 117-19, *118*, *119*, 151; demand 118; fixed-rate 118; natural (sino-atrial node) 23, *23*, 25, 76, 117; temporary 122, *129*
Paget, Stephen 13-14
palpation 73
palpitations 71, 141
paroxysmal nocturnal dyspnoea 71
Patel, Chandra 170
patent ductus arteriosus 26-7, 56, 61-2, *62*
pectin 95
pericardium *17*, 58
personality 166-7
phenytoin 94
'piggy back' transplants 110
pituitary gland 158
plaque *65*, 66, 85, 99, 147
plasma 20
platelets (thrombocytes) 20, 66, 85, 86, 148, *148*, *149*, 200
pneumonia 71
Pomerance, Ariela 112
potassium 90, 94
pregnancy 49, 50-52, *50*, 91

Priminger, Paul 95
procainamide 94, 128
processed foods 140, 143, 155, 198; *see also* junk food
propranolol 90
prostacyclin 148, *148, 149*
prostaglandins 148
prosthetics *see* spare parts
proteins 199
pulmonary artery *see* arteries
pulmonary atresia 62
pulmonary circulation *see* blood circulation
pulmonary stenosis *see* stenosis
pulmonary valve *see* valves
pulmonary veins *see* veins
pulse: pressure 158; rate 26, 204-205; taking 205; *see also* heartbeat
pumps 150-51
P waves *77*

Q

quality of life 43, 111
quinidine 94
Q waves *77*

R

radioisotopes 78, *81*
Rahe, R. 160, 161-2
rauwolfia compounds 142
Rehn, Ludwig 14, 15
rejection 40-41, 42, 44, 105, 110-11, 112, 146
relaxation 168, 170-79; progressive 173-4; *see also* meditation
revascularization 150
rheumatic fever 99, 146
rheumatic heart disease 25
rhythmodan 94
Rodin, Judith 193, 194-5
Roscuer, Andreas *13*
Rosemann, Ray 166
rubella 50-51
R waves *77*, 105

S

Saint, Charles 48
Saint Jude valves 99
salt 93, 140, 143, 198
Sargant, William 166
Sauerbruch, Ferdinand 102
scanning *see* ultrasound scanning
screen oxygenator *33*
self-healing mechanisms 148
self-help groups 136, 197
Selye, Hans 166
septa 18, 55, 58
septal defects 55-9, 78; atrial 56, *56*, 58-9, 78; ventricular 55-6, *56*, 58, 60, 61, 62
sex 98, 135
Shackleton, Ernest 157
shock *122*
Shumway, Norman 41, 42
'shunts' 55-6, 58, 60, 61, 78
Shute, Wilfred E. 94-5
side-effects 142; anticoagulants 92; beta

blockers 91; digitalis 89-90; diuretics 94; nitrates and nitrites 90; rhythm-controlling drugs 94; sleeping tablets 179
sino-atrial node *see* pacemaker (natural)
sleep 143, 178-9
smoking 66, 82, 83, 85-6, 122, 131, 141, 142, 146, 155, *181, 187*; pregnancy and *49*, 50, 52; reasons for 182; restarting 187; staying stopped 187; stopping 136, 143, 180-87
smoking diaries 181, 186
social-readjustment rating scale 160-62
soldier's heart 71, *72*
Souttar, Henry 16
spare parts (prosthetics) 44-6; *see also* heart (artificial); pacemaker (artificial)
spasm 149
Speilberger, Charles 169
sphygmomanometers 138-9, 140
Stark, Jaroslav 63
Starr, Albert 46
Starr–Edward valve 101
Starr valve 46, 99
starvation diet 197
stenosis 25, 59; aortic *59*; mitral 16, 59, *59*, 99; pulmonary 59-60
stethoscope 73, *73*, 74
streptococci 25
streptokinase 92, 150
stress 82, 141, 155; causes 157-8; checking 164-5; countering and controlling 143, 156-79; effects 158-9; job-stress 162-5, 170; responses to 167-9; smoking and *187*; testing *158*
stress hormones *see* adrenalin
stroke (cerebral haemorrhage) 66, 136, 138, 147
sugar intolerance *see* glucose intolerance
superior vena cava *17*
surgery *see* heart surgery; obesity (surgery and)
'Surveyor' monitors 147
Survivors Trial 130-31
S waves *77*
sweating, excessive 142
swelling *see* oedema
symptoms 69-72, 73; of hypertension 138, 141-2, *142*
syphilis 25, 99, 103
systemic circulation *see* blood circulation
systole 22
systolic pressure *see* blood pressure

T

tachycardia 26, 76
Teflon 44, 59
telephone pacemaker checks 118-19, *119*
Tenormin (atenolol) *91*
Tetralogy of Fallot 59-61, *59, 60, 61*
thalidomide 51
Thelle, Dag 85
thiazides 93-4
thrombocytes *see* platelets
thromboses *see* clots
thrombosis, coronary 25, 92, 94, 121
thromboxane 148

thyroid gland 194
Timson, Edward *98*
tissue-matching 44
tissue-typing 103, 110
TM (transcendental meditation) *see* meditation
transplantation 29; *see also* heart transplants; kidneys (transplants)
transvenous implantation 118
tricuspid atresia 62
tricuspid valve *see* valves
tuberculosis 65
Tuffier, Dr. 15
tumours 48, 102, 140
T waves *77*
Type A people 166-7, *166*
Type B people 166-7

U

UCT valve 101
ulcers: peptic 103; stomach 35
ultrasound scanning (echocardiography) *50, 51*, 52-3, *52*, 78-80, *81, 82*, 147
urination 93-4

V

vagus nerve 89
valves 99-101; aortic *17*, 18, 19, *25*, 99; artificial 44-6, 92, 99-101, *100, 101, 102*; biological replacement 101; blocked 150; damaged 136; deformities 15, 25; diseases affecting 25; mitral 16, *17*, 18, 59, 99, *100*; narrowed 15; operations on 15, 16, 96, 99-101, *100*; pulmonary *17*, 18, 19, 60, 61; sounds associated with *73*, 74; tricuspid *17*, 18, 19; *see also* stenosis
valvotomy 61
valvuloplasty 150
vascular disease 103
vasoconstriction 103, 148
vasodilation 143, 148, 149
veins 19, *19*; pulmonary *17*, 19
ventilators, mechanical 128; *see also* lungs (artificial)
ventricles 18, *77*, 128; aneurysm of 102; left *17*, 19, 82; right *17*, 19, 55-6
ventricular septal defects *see* septal defects
verapamil 94
viral infections 24, 50-51, 99, 145, 146
virology 145
vitamins 95, *201*; A 85; C 95; E 94-5

W X Y

Wade, John 106-109
warfarin 92
Washkansky, Louis 42, *43*
water, hard 82, 95
weight control *see* obesity (control)
Weightwatchers 197
Weyrauch, Frank 63
Withering, William 89, *89*
work: job-stress 162-5, 170; return to after heart attack 134-5
X-rays 74, *74*, 76, 78
Yacoub, Magdi 106, 108, 112

Acknowledgements

A book, like a heart operation, is the result of teamwork and co-operation. Many people contributed to the making of this book, and we sincerely thank them.

Dr. Paul Curry of the Cardiac Department at Guy's Hospital, London, commented on the typescript and provided extra words on emergency and drug treatment of heart failure; Dr. David N. McVerry contributed additional material to the heart transplantation section and also checked the captions; Paul Barnett copyedited the book and prepared the index; Dr. Phil Whitfield, of Kings College, University of London, cast an expert eye over the more complex illustrations; and Papworth Hospital, England, provided details of the Papworth method of heart transplantation.

For permission to quote excerpts we would like to thank: J.J. Lynch, *The Broken Heart*, Basic Books, 1978 (*pages 86 and 87*); *The Sunday Times* (*page 112*); T. Holmes and R. Rahe, 'The Social Readjustment Scale', in the *Journal of Psychosomatic Research*, vol II, 1967 (*pages 160 to 161*); C.L. Cooper, *The Stress Check*, Prentice Hall, 1981 (*pages 162 to 163*); J. Steinmetz, 'The stress reduction program at University Hospital, University of California Medical Center, San Diego', *Proceedings of the Conference on Occupational Stress*, sponsored by the National Institute of Occupational Safety and Health, November 1977 (*pages 164 to 165*); C. Wood, 'Relax, and stop a heart attack', *New Scientist*, vol. 100, no. 1379, 1983 (*page 168*); Thames Television Limited, *How to Last a Lifetime*, 1981 (*pages 170, 174, 179*); B.B. Brown, *Stress and the Art of Biofeedback*, Bantam Books, 1977 (*pages 171, 172, 173, 174*); R.K. Peters and H. Benson, 'Time out from tension', *Harvard Business Review*, January/February 1979 (*page 172*); The Open University in association with the Health Education Council and the Scottish Health Education Unit, *The Good Health Guide*, Harper and Row, 1980 (*page 182, 186*); M. Polunin (Ed.), *The Health and Fitness Handbook*, Windward and Here's Health, 1981 (*page 184*); J. Rodin, *Controlling Your Weight*, Century, 1983 (*pages 190, 191, 192, 193*).

For their fine draughtsmanship, and for doing what photographs cannot do, our thanks also go to: Frank Kennard (*pages 17, 18, 19, 22, 104, 105*); Sarah Kensington (*pages 124, 125, 206, 207, 208, 209, 210, 211, 212, 213, 214, 215, 216, 217*); Janos Marffy (*pages 21, 27, 32, 33, 37, 56, 60, 62, 65, 68, 70, 77, 83, 96, 100, 137, 185, 205*); Mulkern Rutherford (*page 23*).

Picture Credits

Aspect Picture Library Carolyn Johns 29, 38 bottom left, 57, 157 bottom left, 158 top **Associated Press** 44 **BBC Hulton Picture Library** 38 top **Biophoto Associates** 24 top left, top right, centre, 26, 67, 80, 88, 145 **Anthony Blake Photo Library** 84, 153, 197 bottom, 200-201 bottom **Colorific!** E Ferorelli 113 top, 116 top, 117, 149 bottom, 150-151, Phillip Hayson 147, Dan McCoy/Black Star 144 **Mary Evans Picture Library** 13, 14 centre, 21 top **Goldcrest** David Barlow 25 **Gower Scientific Photos** 52 **Sally and Richard Greenhill** 49, 50, 134, 157 bottom right, 159, 166, 184-185, 187, 195, 196, 199, 203 **John Heseltine** 156, 157 top, 181, 202 bottom, 204 bottom **Illustrated London News Picture Library** 36 **Image Bank** Walter Bibikow 75 left, Gary Bistram 130, Lawrence Fried 14 bottom, Ellis Herwig 128 bottom, 204 top, Lou Jones 171, Barbara Kreye 188, P O Malibu 132, Marc St. Gil 55 bottom, 176, Zao-Grumberg 178, Zao-Longfield 174-175 **Camilla Jessel** 53 bottom, 55 top **Anthony McCormack** 53 top, 189 **Mansell Collection** 12 **Multimedia Picture Library** 177, 193, 194, John Heseltine 90, 91, 93, 94 **Museum Boerhaave, Leiden** 39 top **The Photosource** Central Press 45, Keystone 30, 41 bottom, 63, 81 top right, 98-99 **The Photographers Library** 133, 141, 201 top right, 204 centre **Rex Features** Sipa Press 47, 113 bottom **Dr J Reidy/Guys Hospital** 9, 64, 74, 79, 82, 100 top right **Ann Ronan Picture Library** 39 bottom, 89 **Science Photo Library** 100 bottom, 101, 102 top and centre, 116 bottom, 119 bottom, 146 **Seaphot/Planet Earth Pictures** Cameron Read 31 **Frank Spooner Pictures** Gamma 34, 114-115 **John Watney Picture Library** 20, 38 bottom right, 41 top, 58, 59, 66, 72, 76, 92, 97, 118, 119 top, 120, 122, 123, 126-127, 129, 131, 138, 139, 142, 158 bottom, 168, 197 top left and top right, 202 top **The Wellcome Foundation Limited** 148, 149 top left and top right **Wellcome Institute Library, London** 14 top, 15, 73 top **Westminster Hospital** 61 **Ian Yeomans/The Sunday Times, London** 106-109, 112 **Zefa** 28, 48, 51, 54, 75 right, 81 top left, centre and bottom, 102 bottom

Multimedia Publications (UK) Limited have endeavoured to observe the legal requirements regard to the suppliers of photographic materia